Praise for *Bedlam's D*

"*Bedlam's Door: True Tales of Madness and Hope* contains fourteen remarkable stories—they are truly turnkey experiences. Sober, riveting, and at times humorous, they are full of surprises. The book provides so much to learn no matter how much you already know about psychology and human behavior."

> —Warren Tanenbaum, MD, Clinical Associate Professor of Psychiatry, Emeritus, State University of New York Downstate Medical Center

"Alas, there is an art to medicine! Mark Rubinstein's *Bedlam's Door* offers a deeply compassionate portrayal of that state of being that transcends normal: madness. The stories are rich, vibrant, surprising, and most importantly, human. Whether you've ever been a psychiatric patient or know someone who has—this book is a must-read!"

> —Helen M. Farrell, MD, Psychiatrist and Forensic Psychiatrist, Harvard Medical School, and Instructor, Beth Israel Deaconess Medical Center

"The stories in *Bedlam's Door* are Mark Rubinstein's vivid and finely wrought accounts of his own interactions with men and women who inhabit the world of mental illness. His consistently humane, attentive, and self-reflective narrative provides the key to unlocking our greater understanding and compassion—essential traits for the crucial endeavor of offering the help and hope these people desperately need."

> —Roger Rahtz, MD, Psychiatrist and Psychoanalyst, New York City

"In Bedlam's Door, Mark Rubinstein presents a series of fascinating clinical vignettes from the field of psychiatry. Rubinstein is a brilliant storyteller who entertains and educates the reader in an empathic and compelling fashion. *Bedlam's Door* is a thoughtfully written book that gives the reader a provocative glimpse into a psychiatrist's world."

—Donna Sutter, MD, MPH, Psychiatrist and former Clinical Assistant Professor, Baylor College of Medicine

"Dr. Rubinstein graciously accompanies the reader across the threshold of *Bedlam's Door* to introduce fourteen struggling souls in the grips of mental illness. In doing so, he skillfully helps dispel the mystery and fear that paralyze the mind of the uninitiated."

—Andrea R. Polans, PhD, Clinical Psychologist, former Clinical Instructor, State University of New York Downstate Medical Center

PRAISE FOR MARK RUBINSTEIN'S NOVELS

The Lovers' Tango

"The tension in these pages never lets you go. Rubinstein is a born storyteller. A gripping legal drama powers this novel at a torrid pace. Mark Rubinstein knows that what goes on outside the courtroom is just as important as what happens inside."

—Michael Connelly, bestselling author of the Harry Bosch series

"Mark Rubinstein's *The Lovers' Tango* is a sultry, elegant piece of romantic noir. It has a terrific legal backdrop that merges the tale into a steamy courtroom thriller focusing on human frailty and the limitations of what we see before us."

—Jon Land, USA Today bestselling author of *Strong Darkness*

"Mark Rubinstein is a superb storyteller. His novels tap into the deepest of human emotions."

—Raymond Khoury, bestselling author of the Sean Reilly series

"*The Lovers' Tango* is much more than a riveting courtroom drama. It is a powerful love story that kept me reading long after I should have been in bed."

—Phillip Margolin, *New York Times* bestselling author of *Woman with a Gun*

"In *The Lovers' Tango*, Mark Rubinstein proves that Nicholas Sparks is not the only author who can masterfully blend suspense, tragedy, and romance into a timeless story of love, loss, and the beguiling mystery of memory. Here is a story within a story, all entwined around a pair of lovers locked in a tragic dance. Once it starts, you'll be unable to tear yourself away as you're carried relentlessly forward to the novel's surprising and poignant ending."

—James Rollins, *New York Times* bestselling author of *The Sixth Extinction* and *War Hawk*

Mad Dog House

"I stayed up all night to read *Mad Dog House*. I didn't plan on it, but when I got into it, I couldn't put it down. It was fantastic, riveting, suspenseful, twisting, loving, horrific."

—Martin West, film and television actor and filmmaker

"The characters in *Mad Dog House* are compellingly real. It was a great read!"

—Ann Chernow, artist and writer

"In Mark Rubinstein's *Mad Dog House*, the characters—all well developed and dripping with authenticity—propel the novel along with style and edge-of-your-seat excitement."

—Judith Marks-White, author of *Seducing Harry* and *Bachelor Degree* and columnist, "The Light Touch," *Westport (CT) News*

"*Mad Dog House* is a gripping, harrowing, and provocative psychological thriller, featuring a plot packed with action and intrigue, staggering and brutal twists, and deeply disturbing possibilities. The author has a gift for delivering gut-punching surprises while raising unsettling questions about the basic nature of human beings and the inescapable hold of the past."

—Mysia Haight, www.pressreleasepundit.com

Love Gone Mad

"*Love Gone Mad* is a beautifully crafted suspense novel. The characters are people you care about; the story is fast paced and cleverly plotted."

—Scott Pratt, bestselling author of the Joe Dillard series

"I quickly found myself caught up in *Love Gone Mad*—part love story, part *Halloween*, and part legal thriller."

—Elissa Durwood Grodin, author of *Physics Can Be Fatal*

"Rubinstein's second foray into the fiction arena (after *Mad Dog House*) is an intense thriller that promises readers surprising twists, heart-pounding suspense, and a bird's-eye view into both the mind of a madman and a dizzyingly realistic account of how it feels to be stalked as prey."

—*Library Journal*

Mad Dog Justice

"What price must a man pay for doing a very bad thing for a very good reason? That is the question *Mad Dog Justice* poses, and the answer is written with great skill and creaks with tension and truth."

—Simon Toyne, author of the internationally bestselling Sanctus Trilogy and *The Searcher*

"*Mad Dog Justice* speeds along with more turns than a Vespa cruising through traffic. It's a smart, twisting thriller that grows into the weightier issues of friendship, vengeance, and betrayal."

—Andrew Gross, bestselling author of *Everything to Lose* and *The One Man*

"*Mad Dog Justice* thrums with relentless intensity and suspense. Rubinstein has created a palpable cast of characters who stay with you long after you finish the book."

—Jessica Speart, author of *A Killing Season* and *Restless Waters*

"Reading *Mad Dog Justice* is akin to being on a treadmill that's been programmed to perpetually increase speed until your heart threatens to burst from your chest. The tension in this novel accelerates to breakneck speed, and just when you think you might get a reprieve, Rubinstein shocks you again."

—Joseph Badal, author of *The Lone Wolf Agenda*

Bedlam's Door

Other Books by Mark Rubinstein

Fiction

Stone Soup

Mad Dog House

Love Gone Mad

Mad Dog Justice

The Foot Soldier, a novella

Return to Sandara, a novella

The Lovers' Tango

Nonfiction

The First Encounter: The Beginnings in Psychotherapy
with Dr. William Console and Dr. Richard C. Simons (Jason Aronson)

The Complete Book of Cosmetic Surgery
with Dr. Dennis P. Cirillo (Simon & Schuster)

New Choices: The Latest Options in Treating Breast Cancer
with Dr. Dennis P. Cirillo (Dodd Mead)

Heartplan: A Complete Program for Total Fitness of Heart & *Mind*
with Dr. David L. Copen (McGraw-Hill)

*The Growing Years: The New York Hospital–Cornell Medical Center
Guide to Your Child's Emotional Development* (Atheneum)

Bedlam's Door

True Tales of Madness and Hope

MARK RUBINSTEIN

Thunder Lake Press

Thunder Lake Press
25602 Alicia Parkway, #512
Laguna Hills, CA 92653
www.thunderlakepress.com

Ordering Information
Quantity sales. Special discounts are available on quantity purchases by corporations, associations, and others. For details, contact the "Special Sales Department" at the address above.

Orders by US trade bookstores and wholesalers. Please contact BCH: (800) 431-1579 or visit www.bookch.com for details.

Printed in the United States of America

Cataloging-in-Publication

Rubinstein, Mark, 1942- author.
  Bedlam's door : true tales of madness & hope / Mark
  Rubinstein. -- First edition.
    pages cm
    Includes bibliographical references.
    LCCN 2016946761
    ISBN 978-1-941016-23-7 (pbk.)
    ISBN 978-1-941016-24-4 (ebook)

    1. Mental illness--Popular works. 2. Mental illness
  --Treatment--Popular works. 3. Mentally ill--United
  States--Case studies. 4. Psychotherapy patients--United
  States--Case studies. I. Title.
  RC454.R76 2016   616.89
  QBI16-900011

First Edition

20 19 18 17 16   10 9 8 7 6 5 4 3 2 1

Contents

Foreword

Psychotherapy is both an art and a science. How often we have heard that truism invoked. But in the true tales that follow, this self-evident fact comes alive before our eyes, thanks to the talent and experience of Mark Rubinstein—physician, psychiatrist, forensic expert, and author.

Certain theologians notwithstanding, the ravages of mental illness are real. Anxiety can paralyze, and depression can morph into despair. Madness destroys reality, and revenge destroys love. Substances burn out the brain, and mania cripples creativity. The experienced therapist meets all these conditions and many more with humility, knowing powerful ghosts from the past live on within each of us, working hard to defeat both the present and the future. Trust and hope can sustain us, but the outcome is never certain.

In *Bedlam's Door* Mark Rubinstein gives many examples of his own psychiatric journey in battling these formidable forces, and they are indeed stories of War ending in varying stages of Peace. They will linger in our memory for a very long time, and we are grateful to him for his courage and his humanity in sharing them with us.

Richard C. Simons, MD
Professor Emeritus of Psychiatry
University of Colorado Health Sciences Center
Past President, American Psychoanalytic Association

Preface

Why would a man of Hungarian descent run down a street ranting "I'm king of the Puerto Ricans"?

Why would a psychiatrically hospitalized young woman sneak a razor blade onto the ward, give it to another patient, and direct her in slitting her wrists?

Why would a woman present herself to surgeons for a dozen operations when nothing is physically wrong with her?

Though they read like fiction, these stories are true. The patients were people my colleagues and I saw in psychiatric consultation or for treatment.

To preserve the anonymity of everyone involved, many particulars have been changed. At times I've created composites, rather than describe one person or incident. Names, dates, locations, and other circumstantial details have been altered. The entity I've called Manhattan Hospital is a conglomeration of the facilities where I worked as a medical student, an intern, a resident, a private practitioner, a teacher, and an attending psychiatrist.

Though quite diverse, these stories have an overarching unity: while they describe different people with varying histories and circumstances, the patients' clinical presentations funnel down to the basic elements of human functioning—how people think, feel, and behave. These tales demonstrate that nearly all mental illness—whether brought about by nature, nurture, or a combination of the two—can be understood when attention is paid to the stories told.

The collection depicts the challenges mental illness poses to patients, their families, and the people charged with their care. It also highlights our country's pressing need to improve mental health care delivery, along with describing the life-altering advances being made in the diagnosis, treatment, and prevention of psychiatric conditions.

Of all medical specialties, psychiatry involves exploring people's lives. One hundred people suffering from a similar condition (for instance, depression) will have one hundred *different* stories to tell. Each case is a minibiography revealing the circumstances and conflicts leading to symptoms. Above all, psychiatry has a *human* dimension, and each patient has a compelling story to share, one that's unique but at the same time taps into a shared commonality.

Whether a story in this collection concerns a prison inmate, a carpenter, a homemaker, a police officer, a short-order cook, a student, or a private investigator, a story of conflict and struggle emerges.

Most of all, these tales depict the humor, sadness, nobility, poignancy, and richness of our human experience.

Mark Rubinstein, MD

No excellent soul is exempt from a mixture of madness.

—ARISTOTLE

King of the Puerto Ricans

"How dare you treat me this way!" boomed a husky voice with a thick Eastern European accent. "I'm king of the Puerto Ricans," came the roar from the packed waiting room.

It was a warm, humid June evening, about eight p.m. Although I'd been a resident for only a few months, my instincts told me this would be one of those nights when the emergency room would earn its moniker as *Bedlam's Door*, a revolving carousel of psychosis, with one disturbed person after another being steered to the facility by the police, family members, or friends.

"King of the Puerto Ricans," bellowed the man, his voice reverberating through the corridor. The claim was utterly absurd—from his self-proclaimed royalty to his non-Hispanic accent. It was bizarre, even for the environs of Manhattan Hospital's emergency room.

Another leonine roar of Slavic-sounding speech brought me to my feet.

Peering into the reception area, I saw a burly man bound securely to the confines of a high-backed wooden wheelchair.

Despite his raging, the man—appearing to be in his sixties—had a cherubic-looking face, with round, rosy cheeks and bushy, dark eyebrows. A huge mane of white hair crowned his head. Highly agitated, he struggled against the canvas straps binding him to the wheelchair. Though his ankles were secured to the contraption's front rigging, he managed to kick and stomp his feet on the footrest.

"Let me go. I have work to do," he roared.

His words were barely comprehensible, partly due to his agitation, but also because he lapsed into a foreign language—perhaps Polish, or some other Slavic-sounding tongue. He shook the wheelchair violently, attempting to break free. A woman wearing a drab housedress tried to quiet him, but he kept shouting.

A police officer I knew saw me and approached.

"What's up, Officer Romano?" I asked.

"He was running down Delancey Street, tossing trash baskets and shouting. We couldn't control him. He's as strong as an ox. You hear what he's yelling?" Romano shook his head. Over the years, he'd brought his share of patients to our doors, but this one clearly perplexed him.

That week I'd already encountered the putative son of God, an enraged Moses, and Satan himself. But I never imagined meeting the king of the Puerto Ricans.

"Who's the woman?" I asked.

"His wife. She said his name's Nathan . . . Nathan B."

"Any previous history you know of?" I asked.

"Nope. The neighbors say he's always been a quiet guy and a hard worker. A carpenter."

A carpenter? Why doesn't he think he's Jesus?

Romano looked at me with raised eyebrows. "You're not gonna give us trouble with this one, are you, Doc?"

He knew I'd sent the police packing scores of times with drunken and disorderly miscreants they dragged to the emergency room, trying to avoid tossing them into the precinct's drying-out tank. The cops hated babysitting drunks almost as much as they loathed the paperwork involved.

But Nathan B. was a man lost in the throes of madness.

"Looks like you're safe on this one, but let me talk to his wife."

Sarah B.'s pale face sagged. Her gray hair was tied back in a bun. She dabbed at her reddened eyes with a handkerchief. In the housedress, she looked like a Russian or Polish peasant woman from a bygone era.

"Mrs. B., how did this start?"

"It was maybe two weeks ago, Doctor," she said with a thick accent. "After Nathan hurt his back."

"What happened?"

"He's a carpenter and was working on the roof of a house. He fell down onto a pile of wood. He's lucky to be alive," she said, again dabbing at her eyes. "He broke a bone in his back, and now he can't work. Maybe never . . . Only if it heals, the doctors said. And they don't know—a man his age. He's sixty-four. And, all he knows is work."

"What happened after the accident?"

"After he got out of the hospital, he was very quiet. He talked to no one—not even me. He just looked out the window. He wasn't my Nathan anymore."

"What do you mean?"

"He seemed so sad, so depressed," she said, brushing away a tear.

"Did he ever have an episode like this before?" I asked, wondering if Nathan B. might be suffering from bipolar disorder.

"No. Never. But after he got hurt, he began talking to himself—strange words. And then came dreams, terrible dreams. He would cry out in his sleep. And when he woke up, he would shake and be covered in sweat. He was so wet, I had to change the sheets. He would pace all night, like a wild beast. And talking to himself—under his breath, in Hungarian. I tell you, Doctor, we never talk in that language . . . only English.

"I asked him, 'Nathan, what's wrong?' and he said, 'I have nightmares.' But he would tell me nothing more. He said, 'Sarah, you would not want to know.'

"It got worse. He would never leave the house." Her lips trembled. "When he heard sirens, he shook. He thought they were coming for him."

"The police?"

"Yes. He said, 'They're coming for me.'"

"Did he tell you why?"

"He wouldn't say. He never did a thing wrong in his life." Tears spilled from her eyes. "I know it's from his life in Europe."

"What happened?" I asked, fairly certain of the events to which she was referring.

"The Nazis," she murmured, as her hands went to her face and she sobbed.

"Mrs. B., where are you from originally?"

"We're from Hungary."

"When did you come to the United States?"

"We came in 1947, after the war."

"Where were you during the war?"

"Nathan lived through Auschwitz. But he never talks about it."

"And what about you? Were you in the camps?"

"No. I lived with a family on a farm. And I met Nathan after liberation."

"In a displaced persons camp?"

She nodded. "And we came here. We made a good life together."

When Nathan was wheeled into the office, his eyes bulged and his face shone with sweat. His shirt was soaked with perspiration. He was restless and his eyes darted from the walls to the ceiling.

I introduced myself, saying, "I'd like to talk with you."

No response. He seemed lost in some inner world.

He wore work pants, heavy boots, and a short-sleeved work shirt. His chest was broad and powerful-looking. His hands, large and roughly calloused, were those of a man who'd done carpentry all his life. His forearms, strapped to the wheelchair's armrests, looked as though cables were bundled within them. A series of blue-black numbers was tattooed on his left forearm—a remnant of Auschwitz.

"Mr. B.?"

"How can you do this?" he growled. Suddenly, his eyes crawled over me. Spittle formed at the corners of his mouth.

"Do what?"

"How dare you tie up a *king*!" he shouted hoarsely.

"How did you become king?"

"God made me king. Do you question his word?" His chin quivered.

I said nothing.

"*Answer* me," he demanded. "Do you question God's word?"

He trembled so intensely, the wheelchair shook.

"No. I don't question God or his word," I said. "But why king of the Puerto Ricans?"

"Such a poor people . . . and persecuted. They must go to their own land." His eyes roamed about the office once again. "What is this place?" he demanded.

"You're at Manhattan Hospital."

"What am I doing here? I'm not crazy."

"You were running down the street, throwing trash cans . . ."

"I was calling my people . . . my subjects."

"What did you have in mind?"

"We must leave before the SS gets here."

"What makes you think they're coming?"

His face tightened, and sweat dribbled from his hairline. "Can't you *see*? There's no time left."

"Before what happens?"

"We'll be taken away . . . to the camps. They want to kill all of us."

"Kill who?"

"My people. All the Puerto Rican people. It will be a holocaust."

"Why now?"

"The time has come."

His eyeballs rolled upward and he fixed his stare at the ceiling. He began muttering a goulash of English, German, and Hungarian.

Nathan B.'s mane of white hair, coupled with his upward gaze, reminded me of Renaissance paintings depicting ancient prophets—maybe something by Caravaggio—painted in dusky colors with ethereal light radiating from some godly presence.

"Mr. B., I understand you began feeling bad a few weeks ago . . ."

His garbled muttering continued. He was lost in a world of messianic revelation. The extent to which deluded thinking could seize a person never failed to amaze me.

I tried again to get him to talk. "I'm king of the Puerto Ricans" was all he would say in English.

"Mr. B., I'm going to admit you to the hospital," I finally said.

His incantations stopped. He turned to me, his eyes burning with pious fury. "You want to make me a slave, so I will work for you."

"You won't be a slave," I said. "You'll be here until you calm down."

"You *Nazi*. God will make you pay for this."

I'd tapped into his past—and the source of his madness.

Nathan was admitted to the fourth-floor men's ward. On the admission form, I wrote "physical examination deferred," certain his agitation would have caused a blood pressure reading of stratospheric heights. It was far more important to sedate him and arrange for the physical examination to be done later. I wrote orders for blood to be drawn when he was calmer—to rule out blood, kidney, or liver problems that could possibly be causing his disordered mental state.

I telephoned the ward and arranged to become Nathan B.'s primary therapist.

I spoke again with Mrs. B. and learned more about Nathan's background. But rather than jump to conclusions, I knew it would be better to let him reveal as much as he would about himself over the course of time. You can never learn all you need to know in one or two sessions with a patient, even if you're certain of the diagnosis.

And, in some crucial ways, a diagnosis may be secondary. Far more important in a case like Nathan's—one involving the acute onset of madness—would be an understanding of his story, by learning the trajectory of his life.

A patient's story is organic—it courses through his being. His secrets would likely be the key to his madness.

By the next day the medication we had given him had dampened his agitation—somewhat. His blood work was normal, with no evidence of a metabolic aberration causing Nathan B.'s mad odyssey through the streets. Dressed in hospital pajamas, he sat in my office near the ward's dayroom.

"Who are you?" was his first question.

I gave him my name and asked if he remembered me.

"No." His eyes narrowed.

"I admitted you here."

"Am I a prisoner?"

"No . . ."

"Then I'm free to leave . . ."

"Well, not really," I said, realizing I'd walked into a trap of my own making.

"I won't build you anything," he seethed, crossing his forearms over his chest.

"Build anything? What do you mean?"

"No bookshelves, no cabinets or furniture. I will build you *nothing*." He thrust his chin forward.

"You don't have to build a thing, Mr. B. And when you're feeling better, you'll be free to leave."

His response was to stare out the window.

By the sixth session in the same cramped office, he was considerably calmer. His hair was neatly combed and he wore street clothing. His voice was no longer hoarse.

"So what do you want to know from me?" he asked. His bushy eyebrows rose and his voice held no trace of belligerence.

"What happened that led to your being hospitalized?"

As I asked the question, an esteemed mentor's words came back to me: *No matter what is said, a patient can never really change the subject. It lurks beneath the surface, ready to emerge.*

He meant there's a driving force in a patient's inner life: a host of feelings and behaviors orbiting around a single issue. And it may emerge in the form of a mental illness.

Nathan sighed. "It's a long story . . ."

"I have time."

"I don't like talking about it."

"I'd like to hear about you."

He peered down at his hands. "You know, I'm a carpenter." He looked up at me and added, "Jesus was a carpenter."

"Yes, but we're talking about you now," I said, wondering if this was a residue of grandiosity—from the king of the Puerto Ricans to Jesus.

"I was an apprentice when I was eight years old. It's all I ever did . . . woodworking and carpentry."

"It's a valuable skill."

"It saved my life," he whispered. Tears shivered in his eyes.

"How?" My curiosity was definitely piqued.

"I was born in a small village a few kilometers north of Budapest." He inhaled deeply, his breath sounding like a bellows releasing air. Tears slithered down his cheeks. "There was my mother, my father, two sisters, and a brother. My grandparents, aunts, and uncles lived there, too." His hands were clasped so tightly, his knuckles turned white.

"Poor is what we were—all of us—but we were happy. My father drove a truck. My mother worked in a knitting mill. When I was thirteen, I was what you call here a master carpenter—a cabinetmaker. I could build anything, for the most beautiful homes. Rich people—Jews and gentiles—would ask for Nathan the carpenter."

I nodded, implicitly asking him to tell me more.

"When I was seventeen, everything ended." His shoulders hunched, a surefire sign of tension. "The SS came in Jeeps and trucks, men with machine guns and rifles. They went through the village—tore up everything—and pushed the Jews into the town square. We took maybe small suitcases, nothing else."

"Yes . . ."

"They drove us away . . . to another town. They took us from all the villages to this place. Hundreds of people were there, just waiting at a train station. It was so cold, my feet had no feeling. But worse was the fear."

I waited for him to continue.

"You've heard of Auschwitz and Birkenau?"

"Yes, of course."

My throat tightened.

"We were taken there—in cattle cars."

I nodded again, not wanting to interrupt him.

"We were squeezed in, standing, pressed together, old people, mothers, fathers, children, babies. It was dark and freezing cold. The old ones died on the train. Babies, too. I cannot tell you the horror of it . . . the moaning, the crying . . . how the train went on and on, the darkness, the smell of it, people groaning, coughing, and dying.

"And when we got there—to Auschwitz—we stood on the train platform. Hundreds of us, shivering and frightened. They separated us. Men on one side, women on the other. Like cattle. A doctor picked out the sick ones, and they were led away. Then an SS officer went down the line of men and asked who had a skill, any skill. Men said they could do one thing or another, but he didn't care if you were a tailor, or a butcher, or if you sold clothing.

"My father stood next to me. It tears my heart out to think of him. He poked me in the back before the officer came to me. This SS officer stopped in front of me and asked, 'What can you do?'

"'I'm a carpenter,' I said."

Nathan swallowed hard and continued. "He nodded, and then he smiled. It was an evil smile. He pointed with his thumb to some men standing at the end of the platform."

Tears rolled down his cheeks.

"They put us to work."

Nathan's hands balled into huge fists.

"That was the last time I saw my family."

Tears hung at the edge of his chin and then fell to the floor.

"I stayed alive because of the work. I built barracks for people who would come on more trains and work and starve, and work more, and then, when they could work no more, they would die in the gas chambers. We worked day and night, in the cold. We slept on top of one another, with men coughing, spitting up blood, and some dying.

"To eat, we had one bowl of soup a day. It was mostly water. I got weaker every day. Others were too weak to go on, so the guards shot them. I knew I could last maybe another month before I would be too weak and be shot or go to the gas chambers."

He paused and stared out the window. Then he turned to me.

"One day I heard two SS officers talking. I knew enough German to understand. They needed cabinets in their barracks. I was very frightened—shaking began in my legs—because we were not allowed to talk to the guards. You could be shot. But I would die soon anyway, so I took a chance.

"I went to them. One pulled his pistol from the holster. I said, 'I can build them for you.' My German was poor, so I moved my hands, like I was using a hammer and saw. They laughed. I thought the guard would shoot me. I was shivering from the cold and from fear.

"But they got another guard who spoke Hungarian. I said, 'I can build you cabinets. I am a master carpenter.'

"They were excited; then the one who spoke Hungarian said, 'We'll see if you lie,' and they took me to their quarters.

"So I became their carpenter. I built cabinets, tables, and bookshelves—whatever they wanted. They had beautiful wood— cherry, mahogany, and ash. I stayed warm in the woodshop—not in the cold like the others. I was making furniture for the SS. They liked my work and fed me well.

"I made gifts for their wives or girlfriends. Carpentry kept me warm; it fed me and kept me alive until liberation."

"And your family?"

"Gone. In the gas chamber, the ovens." He shuddered. "There was smoke from the crematorium, and I knew they were there, in that smoke going up to the sky. My mother and father, my sisters and brother, everyone—all burned. I could smell them in the air. And I thought maybe I could see them in the smoke. The sky was dark with ash." He shook his head as tears streamed down his cheeks. "How can I describe the horror of the camp . . . a place of corpses, gas, and ashes?"

I shivered at the image Nathan's words evoked.

"And what was I doing? Eating good food, sleeping in a warm bed, alive and working for the SS."

"Yes, you lived . . ."

"Because of these hands," he muttered, staring at them.

"How did that make you feel?"

He said nothing, just sat amid his sadness.

We remained silent for what seemed a long time.

"And after liberation?" I asked.

He looked up. His bleary eyes swerved to me. "I was in a camp for the homeless. I was twenty years old. I had nobody. Not a soul in the world. Everyone I loved . . . all dead. The camp was where I met Sarah. And we came here—where we could live like people, not animals."

"What happened then?"

"In America, I got a job as a carpenter. And I learned English."

"Tell me, Nathan, did you think about your family? Did you cry for them?"

He shook his head. "I stayed busy with my work—with these hands." He sighed, averting his eyes.

"The hands that kept you alive?"

"Yes."

"Do you have children?"

"No. It was not to be. We take what this life gives us. You just live the best way you can."

"After you got here, did you think about the camp?"

"Never. We had a new life here. Just Sarah and me and the work."

Shuddering began in his shoulders.

"What's wrong?" I asked.

"Nothing," he whispered, staring downward.

"It doesn't look that way."

His eyes rose to meet mine. "I would be fine if I could be a carpenter again."

"It was when you hurt your back that this trouble began?"

He looked away.

"That's when the dreams began, right?"

He turned chalky white. His lips trembled.

"Tell me the dreams."

"It was horrible . . ."

He'd said "it." He hadn't used the plural "they."

"What was horrible?"

"The camp. That place . . ."

"Is that what you dreamed about?"

He nodded.

"And the dreams began after you were hurt?"

"Yes."

He fell silent.

Had I pushed too hard, too fast? Had I broached his past too quickly? Had I picked at the scabs of his wounds too soon? He might become agitated again and try to redress the wrongs in his life. It might be better to end the session rather than to let him talk more about Auschwitz.

I waited, not sure what to say or do.

But then he looked at me in the strangest way. The skin around his eyes tightened.

"You have no idea what it was like . . ."

I nodded, understanding his meaning.

"If you live a thousand years, you should never see what I saw."

"The horror of Auschwitz," I said in a near whisper.

"Auschwitz and the dreams." Tears dripped to the floor. "I never dreamed of it in all the years after liberation. I kept it from my thoughts. But then it all came back—forty years later. It came alive, like it happened yesterday."

"Can you tell me the dream?"

He locked his eyes onto mine. "In the dream, I'm back there—at Auschwitz, with my tools, going to the workshop to make furniture and gifts. The wind blows and the sky is dark. The prisoners are in rows . . . starving, standing on dead feet. Some are shot through the head—one by one—men and women. The children are already dead. Dogs are barking—vicious beasts with wet teeth. If you don't obey, the guards let the dogs tear you apart.

"The bodies are piled high, near pits; hundreds and hundreds of naked corpses on top of one another. And there are mounds of shaved hair, mountains of suitcases and clothing, shoes stacked as high as your shoulders, and lines of naked men and women being whipped and pushed to the gas chambers.

"The dead are thrown into wheelbarrows—their arms and legs hang over the sides and swing like toy dolls. They wheel them to the crematorium to be burned, to turn into cinders. Death, disease, and starvation are everywhere. The lucky ones never live more than a day in the camp.

"The air is filled with smoke and the smell of burning flesh, and the sky turns green and black. When the wind blows, ash goes in my mouth and nose. I try not to breathe, but maybe they are the ashes of my mother, or my father's flesh, or that of my sisters or brother, and I can breathe them in, and if I take the air in—I can have them with me once more.

"You can smell it for miles," Nathan said in a trembling voice. "I cover my eyes and nose with a rag, but there's no escape from it. It's the smell of death. There's shouting in German and Polish and Hungarian, and the barking dogs, and the people crying and moaning, going to the gas chambers.

"But not me . . . the carpenter, the one the Germans loved because of these hands."

"And this is what you see in your dreams?"

"I see it . . . every night. After forty years with no dreams, it all came back."

"The dreams," I said tentatively. "You never had them before you hurt your back?"

"No. Never before. I was living a normal life—like it never happened. That's all I wanted in this life, to live and be left alone."

He sighed.

"I just wanted to make a new life with Sarah, here in America."

"And . . . ?"

"I *had* to forget. I used these hands, and I worked and worked, and never stopped."

"Do you think you forgot your past?"

He shook his head. "It's all back now, like it was yesterday."

"It was never gone," I said.

He gazed into my eyes. "It's—it's such a terrible thing, the past. It hangs around my neck like a stone."

"Your past life . . . ?"

"Yes. And the anger I feel."

I nodded.

"This bitterness . . . it eats at me. It's . . . it's . . . I cannot describe it." He peered out the window and then turned to me. "If I could tear open my chest, and if you could lick my heart, it would poison you."

A lump formed in my throat.

"And now it's all back," he whispered.

"The past never dies," I said.

"The poison came out." He closed his eyes and clasped his hands.

"So, Nathan, do you remember running down the street and shouting you were king of the Puerto Ricans?"

"I have some memory of it."

"Do you know why that happened?"

"I wanted to save them. I was crazy."

"Maybe *it* was crazy, but *you* aren't crazy. I think you understand what happened now."

Tears shimmered in his eyes. "It was after I hurt my back, yes?"

"When you could no longer be a carpenter."

He shook his head.

"It's what held you together . . . from Auschwitz until now. The wood, the hammer, and the nails."

"So what do I do now?"

"We don't know yet. Your back could heal."

"And if it doesn't?"

"There's woodwork with smaller things. Not houses."

"Will it be enough?"

"We'll see. Along with some medicine—at least for a while. And if we keep talking about what poisoned you—the things you've held in—I think you'll feel better."

"I can't hold this in my heart anymore."

"It would be better to talk about it."

"Will I still see you?"

"We can arrange that."

"Nathan B. survived the concentration camp because of his skilled hands," I said to Dr. Conway, my supervising psychiatrist.

"But the horror smoldered inside him," Conway said.

"It took forty years to surface."

"Yes, it lay dormant," he replied. "And it erupted when he could no longer work. I must confess, in all my years of practice, I've only seen two cases of delayed-onset post-traumatic stress disorder. This is the second one . . . but it was delayed by forty years."

"But king of the Puerto Ricans? I'm not sure I understand that," I said.

"It was PTSD complicated by psychosis. In his delusion, as king of the Puerto Ricans, he could—in fantasy—*save* people rather than merely survive the terror of his past. He was trying to assuage his guilt for having survived when the others died," Conway said, lighting his pipe.

"And carpentry was the link to his past," I said. "But for as long as he could work, it kept the horrors buried."

"That's right," Conway said. "Carpentry was the outlet valve. It kept his memories in check. But without his craft, the valve was gone, and he was thrown back to the camps, where he relived the horror.

"This man's pathology demonstrates something very important, in psychiatry and in life," Conway said. "You can't just shove the past aside. It stays with you, whether you want to acknowledge it or not." Conway paused and added, "As William Faulkner said in *Requiem for a Nun*, 'The past is never dead; it's not even past.'"

Afterword

Nathan B. continued his treatment in the outpatient clinic. Over the next few months he was able to return to a limited form of carpentry. He no longer worked for the construction company, but instead became a freelance carpenter working from his home.

As when he was a boy, the neighbors knew of his skills and called upon him frequently. They asked him to build small items. Nathan's basement was filled with woodworking equipment. He built mantelpieces, jewelry boxes, birdhouses, chairs, stools, small tables, and cabinets, requiring no heavy lifting, climbing, or strenuous activity.

I saw Nathan once monthly for the next year and maintained him on a small dose of antidepressant medication, which, after six months, was no longer necessary.

The home-based carpentry work was enough to soak up his mental and emotional energy. And as it had done for years, the work reenacted his survival at Auschwitz, but also allowed Nathan to rebury the bitterness in his heart.

What would happen years later when, as a very old man, he could no longer work? Would he again go mad? Or would his newfound understanding enable him to adapt to that stage of life? It was impossible to know.

But for the time being Nathan B. was able to relegate the horror of his past to the darkest recess of his mind and go on with his life in America.

Nathan's story illustrates many things: survivor's guilt, the horror of post-traumatic stress disorder, the strange tenacity of memory, and above all, the enduring power of past experiences on a person's functioning—even on an entire way of life.

It also reveals the Herculean efforts made by a traumatized man not only to suppress the terrors of his youth but to relegate them to the deepest recesses of his mind. Nathan tried valiantly to discard the trauma of Auschwitz, to banish it from consciousness, only to have it resurface hauntingly when his defensive construction—carpentry in America—crumbled.

His illness was a magical attempt to undo his helplessness as a prisoner in Auschwitz. So, in his sick fantasy, he became a "king." In essence, it was a mad reconstruction of his life, a redrawing of his terrifying inner mental and emotional landscapes. His insane dash down the streets of New York, and his grandiose delusion of kingship, were the refuge of last resort, one to which he retreated when his life as a carpenter seemed about to end.

Nathan's madness—a desperate attempt at restoration and redefinition—was a final common pathway for the entire arc of his tragic life.

A Helping Hand

She stood before us, trembling, with her head downcast, eyes closed. Ellen was a frail, twenty-one-year-old woman with long blond hair and delicate features. She had spent a week on the locked women's ward, following an apparent suicide attempt after her boyfriend had ended their relationship. From a bottle containing thirty Valium pills, Ellen had swallowed seven tablets. Her mother had found her unconscious in her bedroom and called 911.

Following a series of evaluations, it was felt Ellen hadn't been truly suicidal, but rather had made a suicidal gesture. After a few days on the locked ward, she was transferred to the open community ward. This was a ward designed for people who, while suffering from a psychiatric condition, were not considered dangerous to themselves or others. The ward provided daily structure; it was not locked; patients dressed in their own clothing and were issued passes on weekends and holidays.

Nineteen other patients, along with the staff, attended the morning meeting held in the dayroom. I was a first-year psychiatric resident assigned to the ward with three other residents. Also present were the attending psychiatrists, psychologists, aides, nurses, and social workers. We were seated in chairs arranged in a circle, when Dr. Butler, the chief attending psychiatrist, introduced Ellen to the group.

A chorus of voices greeted her, but Ellen said nothing. She simply stood in place.

"You look like you could use a roommate," called Gloria, a twenty-three-year-old woman who'd been admitted three weeks earlier. Gloria's roommate had been discharged only two days before, so there was an empty bed in her room. Gloria's statement was a friendly gesture to Ellen, who responded with only a nod, still looking down.

Before being admitted, Gloria had been depressed. She'd resorted to using heroin as her drug of choice, partly to lessen her depressed feelings and also to satisfy the addictive cravings brought on by the drug. She'd been weaned from the opiate and was maintained on a daily dose of methadone.

Ellen took a seat, and the meeting began. The usual topics were discussed: a group trip to a museum, a new pool table for the dayroom, a vote about which movie would be shown Friday evening, and other routine matters affecting life on the ward.

Ellen sat quietly, peering down at her hands. When she looked up, her eyes appeared unfocused. A few attempts were made to draw her out, but she barely responded. Instead she sat quietly, and her eyes brimmed with tears.

Later, the staff met in a conference room to discuss each patient's status. Ellen's attending psychiatrist, Dr. Cynthia Drake, said, "I don't think she intended to kill herself. She took her mother's Valium, knowing her mother was home. There were thirty pills in the bottle and Ellen took only seven."

Everyone agreed Ellen's presumed suicide attempt was basically a gesture—there was very little chance her actions would have, or could have, led to her death. Rather, she took the pills as a "message" to her boyfriend, or perhaps, as a call for help.

Ellen was noted to be a beautiful young woman who, despite her outstanding college grades and accomplishments, was passive and judged her self-worth by whether or not she was accepted by others.

"So she presents with two levels of pathology," said Butler. "There's major depression superimposed on a passive personality with very little self-esteem."

Butler added, "We can get her over the depression—the *state* she's in now—but we can't change her personality style, her basic *traits*. Psychotherapy is useless. The only way to get her out of this state is with medication. After all, we can't do a personality transplant."

Butler always championed a biologic approach to treating mental illness. He viewed medication as the solution to virtually all psychiatric problems. A tension-filled static could sizzle in staff meetings. Butler's strictly biologic approach differed from Drake's. While she acknowledged the powerful influence of biology, Drake felt the effects of early childhood experiences were crucial. In her view, psychotherapy could help people readjust their interpersonal thermostats, resulting in more adaptive behavior.

As a first-year resident, I hadn't formed a firm opinion about the preponderance of biology versus psychology as the basis of mental illness. But there seemed little doubt that patients hearing voices or believing radio waves controlled their thoughts were people whose brain cells were misfiring in an explosion of cerebral confusion. But other issues remained open for discussion—the actual cause or causes of illnesses and the best ways to treat them.

"What about Gloria and Ellen being roommates?" a nurse asked. "Do you think they'll get along?"

"I don't see why not," Butler said. "Gloria got along well with Cyndi when she was here. I don't see why it would be different with Ellen."

"Gloria has a forceful personality," said Drake. "She might be a good influence on Ellen. She also did very well in college, so they might have something in common.

"What do you think of Gloria's offering to be her roommate this morning?"

"It was a gracious thing to say, though it's academic," Butler replied. "The only opening on the ward is that one."

"Speaking of being gracious," Drake interjected, "I find Gloria just a bit too ingratiating, don't you?"

The word *ingratiating* is a loaded one in psychiatry. It's often used to refer to sociopathic people, those who present with antisocial personality disorder. They're manipulative individuals who demonstrate callous disregard for the feelings of others. They lack the capacity to experience guilt and often blame others or offer rationalizations for their maladaptive behavior.

"Maybe Gloria is overly ingratiating, even manipulative," Butler said. "But that's the only open slot. Are you implying she has sociopathic qualities?"

"I'm not sure. She's a complicated woman. I don't think we can label her very easily."

We discussed the fact that Gloria's first weekend pass began the next day. She had been taking methadone regularly, was heroin-free, and it was time for a trial outing back in the world. Ellen would be alone for the weekend until Gloria returned. "It'll be a good transition for her," Butler said.

Everyone agreed.

The dayroom was brightly lit on Monday morning. Patients and staff filtered into the dayroom for the community meeting.

"Where are Ellen and Gloria?" someone asked.

"They were talking after Gloria got back from her pass last night," Mary Doyle, a nurse, said. "They've formed quite an attachment." She stood. "I'll get them." She left the dayroom and headed down the corridor.

"Good morning, everyone," Dr. Butler said to the group.

There was the usual chorus of greetings—some sluggish, others more animated.

"Emergency!" came a cry from the hallway. "Help! Emergency!"

We bolted out of the dayroom and ran *en masse* down the corridor.

"In here!" shouted Mary. Her voice came from the room shared by Ellen and Gloria.

We entered the room. Ellen sat on the bed, leaning against the wall. Her eyes looked empty. Blood leaked from her wrists onto her jeans and the bedding.

She'd slit both wrists.

Rushing to her, we compressed her veins, partly stopping the flow of blood.

"Get her to the general hospital ER, *stat!*" Butler shouted.

An orderly appeared with a gurney, and Ellen was rushed down the hall to the elevator.

A single-edge razor blade lay on the bed in a shimmering puddle of blood.

Using forceps, Mary picked up the blade. "Where'd this come from?"

Gloria sat on her bed, saying nothing.

"Did you bring this onto the ward?" Mary demanded.

Gloria nodded her head.

"Why?"

Gloria shrugged her shoulders.

"Ellen's going to be all right," Butler said, returning to the room. "They're superficial cuts. The bleeding's almost stanched and—"

Seeing the razor blade, Butler stopped talking midsentence. "What's this?" he said.

"Gloria brought *this* back to the ward last night," said Mary.

Butler's mouth opened, but he said nothing.

The silence was dense.

Gloria stared into space.

"Why?" Butler asked. "Why did you bring this here?"

Gloria mumbled something unintelligible.

"What?" Butler demanded. "What're you saying?"

"She wanted help . . ." Gloria said.

"Help?" Butler asked. "Help *killing* herself?"

Gloria looked away.

"So you brought a razor blade back here? *That* was the help you gave her?"

"I was just trying to help her," Gloria said.

The tone of the staff meeting was somber.

"I take full responsibility," Butler muttered. "I can hardly believe this."

"Human behavior is so unpredictable," Drake said, trying to soothe him.

"Is it?" replied Butler. "Only Friday we were wondering if Gloria has sociopathic tendencies."

"Come on, Fred," Drake said. "No one could have foreseen this."

"Gloria's definitely a sociopath," Butler said. "She doesn't belong on this ward."

Drake placed her hand on his arm.

"She actually decided to help Ellen kill herself." Butler shook his head.

"I talked with Ellen at the general hospital," said Drake. "Gloria showed her where to make the cuts."

"Talk about assisted suicide," said a resident.

No one laughed at his attempt at humor.

"Ellen repeated her behavior, right here on the ward," Drake said. "She attempted to commit suicide where help was nearby, just like she did at home with her mother. It was another gesture . . . a cry for help."

We all sat in stunned silence.

Afterword

This brief tale brings certain psychiatric issues into focus.

The first is that even on a hospital ward, where a patient spends twenty-four hours a day, mental health professionals can be fooled by a clever or manipulative patient. This is especially true when someone not only has sociopathic tendencies, but is particularly adept at manipulating others. Correct diagnosis and understanding of the person can be even more difficult when the underlying personality traits are masked by a symptomatic problem, which in this case was Gloria's heroin use.

Someone with antisocial personality disorder is described as presenting with certain characteristic qualities. These usually (but not always) include the failure to conform to social norms, repeated episodes of deception, frequent impulsiveness, aggression (which can take various forms), reckless disregard for the safety of others, irresponsibility, and lack of remorse or rationalization for having mistreated or hurt other people.

It's important to realize that while diagnostic categories have been established for antisocial personality disorder (and all other diagnosable psychiatric disorders), patients may not present with the accepted roster of signs and symptoms. As I like to say, patients *rarely read the textbook* (or *DSM-5*), and their presentations often don't conform to the classical descriptions provided in books.

An important issue brought up by Ellen's situation is that of depression leading to suicide attempts or suicidal gestures.

A few facts about suicide and suicide attempts are worth mentioning. According to the Centers for Disease Control and Prevention, nearly forty thousand Americans managed to kill themselves in 2010. As residents, we learned about gender differences concerning suicide. Four times as many women as men *attempt* suicide, yet four times as many men *succeed* in killing themselves.

The reason, generally acknowledged, is that men's suicidal

behavior is more violent—and effective—than that of women. Men often use guns, jump from high places, and hang themselves—instantly lethal methods with little chance for the person to survive. Women, on the other hand, often attempt suicide by overdosing with pills, turning on oven gas, or slashing their wrists—methods allowing time for lifesaving measures to be taken. Of course, these generalities have many exceptions.

The situation with Ellen was both commonplace (wrist slashing) and unusual (being provided with the means and given instructions by another person).

Gloria was a patient with sociopathic tendencies that were complicated by addictive behavior. After the incident Gloria was viewed as an inappropriate patient for an open community setting. She was discharged from the ward to continue treatment at the hospital's outpatient methadone clinic, where she also received counseling.

Ellen remained on the ward for a few weeks, improved symptomatically, and after discharge, continued in treatment with Dr. Drake.

To the best of my knowledge, Ellen's family never brought a lawsuit against the hospital. Had they done so, they would have likely prevailed in court because of the hospital's failure to carry out its inherent responsibility to protect its patients.

I'll address the issue of legal liability for hospital mishaps or negligence later in this book.

The incident with Gloria and Ellen made such an indelible impression, it motivated me to write an article entitled "Suicide and the Participation of Others,"[1] which was published in the journal *Diseases of the Nervous System*, now known as *The Journal*

---

1. Mark Rubinstein, "Suicide and the Participation of Others," *Diseases of the Nervous System* 37 (September 1976): 534–36.

of Clinical Psychiatry.

No psychiatrist can enter a patient's mind and determine what he or she truly intended at a time of profound despair. Many of us find it difficult to comprehend anguish of sufficient depth to drive someone to the extreme act of ending one's life. Such a desperate act runs counter to the powerful and near-universal instinct for survival.

When assessing suicidal intent, a clinician must depend on training, education, and, above all, experience. In evaluating a patient's propensity for suicide, the clinician must also consider the circumstances in which suicidal behavior may occur.

Suicide attempts have different degrees of severity. Some are invariably lethal, while others fail. But there are no hard-and-fast rules about the seriousness or potential lethality of self-destructive behavior. A gesture may inadvertently succeed, while a serious suicide attempt may fail. Psychiatric journals are filled with clinical anecdotes about people who are viewed, retrospectively, as having made gestures that succeeded. Classically, these involve an overdose of medication in which the person making the gesture was not discovered in time by a family member. As a consequence, the person died from the effects of the drug.

And there are situations where serious attempts have failed.

I recall two patients from my practice who failed in their attempts at suicide.

Lesley and her husband had separated a few months earlier. As a result, she became profoundly depressed. I saw her regularly in psychotherapy sessions, and she took her antidepressant medication faithfully. But it's impossible to know the true depth of depression in another person. So many variables can be in play; the outcome is always shrouded in doubt. A mental health professional must use training, education, and experience in making a considered judgment about the likelihood of a patient's self-destructive tendencies. But it often boils down to an educated estimate, or even a guess. One night, alone in what had once been the couple's apartment, Lesley drank a pint of vodka to dull her psychic pain and lull herself to sleep.

But instead of being a soporific analgesic, the alcohol managed to suffocate any restraint Lesley may have had. It acted as an enabler to her depressive, self-destructive wishes. She flew into a self-directed rage at the misfortunes of her life.

In a state of drunken despair, barely able to maintain physical balance and stumbling about, Lesley taped the apartment windows and door, sealing them off completely. She then staggered into the kitchen and turned on the oven gas, trying to asphyxiate herself.

Luckily, her inebriation caused her to apply the duct tape ineffectively, and the odor of gas seeped out into the hallway. Alarmed neighbors called 911. In a semiconscious state, Lesley was rushed to the hospital, where her life was saved.

This failed attempt could never be regarded as a mere gesture. It was a serious suicidal act, which, fortunately, did not succeed. Lesley recovered and was eventually able to restore her psychic equilibrium and go on with her life.

The other case of a failed but very serious attempt involved Anne, a thirty-year-old, very dependent woman who'd always lived with her parents in their New Jersey home. She worked only occasionally as a "temp" doing filing, never had a serious romantic relationship, and had only a few friends from her high school days whom she rarely saw. She'd never managed to separate from her parents, lived a constricted lifestyle, and failed to form her own adult identity in the world.

Her parents felt the time had come for Anne to get a full-time job and to begin living on her own.

At her first and, as it turned out, only appointment with me, Anne came to my office with her parents, sister, and brother-in-law, all of whom gathered in my consultation room. We discussed the steps she would need to take and the roles her family would play in helping her achieve some modicum of independence.

It was agreed Anne would live temporarily in Manhattan with her sister and brother-in-law while she looked for full-time employment and an apartment near her sister's. She would see me once weekly for psychotherapy sessions while making this transition.

As we talked, I did my best to evaluate Anne in the face of the demands being placed upon her. She was very passive and contributed little to the discussion.

The family left my office.

Alone with Anne, I explored her feelings. Though ambivalent about the proposed arrangement, she expressed willingness to give it a try. My overall impression was she was anxious, not depressed, and emotionally quite immature. Though I had reservations about the potential for success, it seemed Anne might profit from the shift to a more adult lifestyle, coupled with counseling sessions. I also felt the transition, if it could be made successfully, would take quite some time to accomplish.

After the session Anne left the office, presumably to rejoin her sister and brother-in-law at their apartment.

Some hours later I received a call from an intern at Lenox Hill Hospital's emergency room. Instead of going to her sister's apartment, Anne went to the 77th Street subway station of the Lexington line. As the number 6 train barreled into the station, she leaped onto the tracks.

She apparently misjudged the jump and managed to miss the third rail. And miraculously, the incoming train did not roll over her. Anne lost a finger but was otherwise unharmed.

No one could have anticipated this extreme act of self-destruction.

It seemed like a failed attempt, but who can be certain?

Was Anne trying to end her life? Was she attempting to punish her parents for having "abandoned" her? Was it a message or an act of hopeless despair?

Sometimes differentiating between a genuine suicide attempt and a gesture can be very difficult.

Anne was transferred to a New Jersey psychiatric hospital for intensive treatment.

I never saw her again.

I must confess: I was relieved when Anne was hospitalized and when I learned she would return to living with her parents upon discharge. I thought about what had happened the day I met with Anne and her family. Though I'd been careful and had spent a great deal of time with all involved, I couldn't help but imagine the headlines in the local newspapers if Anne had succeeded in killing herself. They would have read something like this: WOMAN LEAVES SHRINK'S OFFICE AND JUMPS TO DEATH.

A *gesture* involves a potentially suicidal act in circumstances where the *actual* risk of death is not substantial, like swallowing too few pills or doing something potentially self-destructive in the presence of others where the chance of being rescued is great.

Suicidal gestures are often viewed as messages to others and may be a depressed person's cry for help. Ellen's slashing her wrists on the psychiatric ward seemed more a gesture than a genuine suicide attempt. The cuts she made were superficial, and she must have known she would be discovered by staff members when she failed to show up at the community meeting.

Ellen's act on the ward was a repetition of what she'd done at home. Recall that before being admitted to the hospital, she took only seven Valium tablets from a bottle containing thirty pills; and she did so while her mother was home and could call for help.

A word of caution is necessary: a depressed person may misjudge things, and a gesture can become mistakenly lethal. And a gesture is always a clear signal of serious psychic pain.

The patient's risk for future suicidal behavior is high and must be evaluated in the context of the person, the family dynamics, other close relationships, and the circumstances in which the presumed gesture occurred.

Nothing in life is completely predictable, none more so than trying to determine a depressed patient's risk for suicide, be it a gesture or a serious attempt.

Virtually anything can happen.

The Head Doctor

As a second-year psychiatric resident, once each week from six p.m. until eight the following morning, I was on psychiatric liaison call. This consultation service provided evaluations for patients who were acting strangely or creating a disturbance in the general hospital. A call would come from a medical or surgical ward, and the psychiatric resident would be dispatched.

One evening, at 10:40 p.m., while sitting in the on-call office glancing through *Sports Illustrated*, I got a call from the charge nurse in the psychiatric emergency room. "Doctor," she said, "a nurse on Surgery Ward 3-B called. A patient is asking for a psychiatric consultation."

"A *patient* wants to see a psychiatrist?"

"That's what she said."

"Did she say it was an emergency?"

"No. Just a consultation."

"Ward 3-B? Surgery?"

"Yes."

"You get the patient's name?"

"No. Just stop at the nursing station and they'll have the information for you."

I got ready to trek to the general hospital, a quarter mile away.

Heading up the emergency ramp of the general hospital, I thought about a consultation on the surgery ward. It was highly unusual for a hospitalized patient to ask for a psychiatric consultation. In fact, it was the first time I could recall it happening. Usually the request came from the medical or nursing staff, not the patient.

When a patient was acting up, an urgent phone call came from a ward nurse or physician. A psychiatrist was needed—immediately. It could be an agitated patient pacing the halls, mumbling incoherently. Maybe it was a side effect of, or an untoward reaction to, a medication. Or someone refusing to take medicine, which could throw the treatment into jeopardy. Sometimes it was a patient demanding to be discharged against medical advice, which could prove dangerous or even life-threatening. The staff wanted to make certain the patient was competent to make such a drastic decision. Or it could be a patient convinced an IV drip contained poison and a murderous conspiracy was afoot.

Usually, a sudden flare-up of uncooperative, odd, or menacing behavior precipitated a request for a consultation.

But this was a very different situation.

A *patient* asking to see a psychiatrist?

Unheard of.

Surgery Ward 3-B was semidark and eerily quiet. It struck me that over one and a half years, I'd grown accustomed to the medley of moans, groans, shrieks, and rantings of a nighttime psychiatric ward. The stillness of a surgical ward seemed utterly foreign. My rubber-soled shoes squeaked on the linoleum floor as I walked along the corridor toward the dimly lit nursing station. Most patients' rooms were darkened; some were lit by bedside lamps. The ward had that antiseptic odor reminiscent of operating rooms, and my thoughts returned to my rotations in general and vascular surgery. I could almost taste the pungency of Betadine on the back of my tongue.

As often happened when I was in the general hospital, I felt estranged from it all. It had been quite some time since I'd been in an OR, assisting with surgery, holding retractors, cauterizing arteries, or working as an intern on a medical ward. The IVs, monitors, and medical paraphernalia seemed part of a past that grew more remote with each passing day.

I had mixed feelings about it: I'd liked surgery and medicine but felt drawn to psychiatry, where every patient's story was unique, often with a deep-seated mystery at the core of the presenting problem. By my third year of medical school—in the middle of the psychiatry rotation—I knew it was the direction my professional life would take.

But there was a downside to my choice: many physicians and nurses viewed psychiatry as a distant and inferior cousin of medicine, not one of the hardcore (read, legitimate) specialties. That attitude of medical superiority was frequently conveyed by staff, sometimes subtly, often openly, when I ventured onto a surgical or medical ward.

And the way psychiatrists dressed in those days didn't do much to bolster our standing in the medical community. Unlike today, when hospital-based physicians of *all* specialties wear white lab coats, back then we psychiatrists dressed in street clothes. My preference was a sports jacket, slacks, and a cloth tie. And there was no stethoscope draped around my neck or protruding from a pocket.

Walking along a corridor in the general hospital, I looked like anything but a physician. I felt light-years removed from physical medicine, even though a mere two years earlier I'd been an intern, elbow-deep in surgeries, delivering babies, drawing bone marrows, starting IVs, and tending to patients in the general hospital.

The nursing station had a long counter behind which the nurses sat doing paperwork. In contrast, the nursing station on a psychiatric ward was set behind wire-reinforced Plexiglas providing an impenetrable protective barrier.

Two nurses were scribbling in patients' charts. It was obvious they were in a hurry. Shift change would occur soon, which meant the departing nurses would "give report" to those arriving, the standard protocol for giving the newly arrived staff a verbal rundown on each patient's status.

I introduced myself. "Someone asked for a consultation . . . ?"

"Oh, yes," said an auburn-haired nurse, rolling her chair toward the rack of patients' charts. "That would be Mr. W. in room 315."

"What's the problem?"

"I have no idea," she said, handing me the chart. "He said he wanted to see a psychiatrist." She resumed writing in a chart.

"And he didn't say why?"

"Not that I'm aware," she replied, never looking up.

It was a curt dismissal.

Sinking into a chair, I opened the chart. I'd long before learned the most revealing entries were made by the nurses—comments about the patient's behavior, complaints about discomfort, notes about sleep patterns, eating habits, restlessness, agitation, or any hint of trouble.

I always saved the nursing notes for last.

For a pleasant change, the surgical entries were easy to read rather than indecipherable doctors' scrawl. The handwritten entries told a clear and simple story.

Calvin W., a forty-three-year-old black man, had been admitted to the hospital for elective surgery. He'd developed an inguinal hernia; a small segment of his large intestine had slipped into the right inguinal canal. Over time the hernia had moved lower into the canal, causing discomfort. The potential danger was the herniated bowel could become trapped in the inguinal canal, cutting off its blood supply. If the bowel segment became strangulated, it could become necrotic—die—and major bowel surgery would be needed to save it.

The protruding segment of bowel slid farther down the inguinal canal, so Mr. W.'s hernia repair had been done. It was a relatively easy procedure, performed routinely in virtually every hospital.

Mr. W.'s temperature chart showed he hadn't developed a fever during his hospital stay, so it was unlikely he was febrile or delirious.

The operative report noted the surgery was done with no complications. Skin to skin in less than forty-five minutes. His time in the recovery room was short and there were no post-op glitches. He'd been transferred to a postsurgical ward bed, to wait one day before discharge.

His medication chart showed he'd asked for Tylenol, nothing stronger. I always reviewed a patient's medications because morphine-based painkillers could cause delirium, slurred speech, slowed thinking, unsteadiness, even hallucinations and a host of behavioral problems. Muscle relaxants, sleeping pills, steroids, and anticonvulsants could also bring on various mental changes.

Despite these possibilities, Mr. W.'s chart revealed nothing problematic.

There was no history of drug or alcohol abuse or psychiatric treatment.

His social history—often given short shrift in hospital charts— revealed he was married and lived in Manhattan with his wife and two kids. He was a short-order cook at a diner on 3rd Avenue and 125th Street, and his wife worked in a bakery.

I turned to the nurses' notes, typically much easier to read than doctors' hieroglyphics. Mr. W. was noted to be calm, cooperative, and resting comfortably at various times during the day, evening, and night. He'd offered no complaints. Soon after the surgery, he was up and about, despite some expectable lower-abdominal pain. He'd advanced from postoperative liquids to a soft diet, and for dinner ate solid food with no problems. There was nothing in the notes about conflicts with nurses or other patients.

But, an entry made at 10:30 that evening written in large and easy-to-read cursive writing, said: "Patient requests psychiatric consultation."

It was signed by J. Lowry, RN.

It was puzzling. The chart profiled a healthy guy who'd come to the hospital for routine elective surgery, nothing more.

So what prompted Calvin W.'s request to see a psychiatrist at 10:30 p.m.?

Slipping the chart back in its rack, I asked, "Is Ms. Lowry around?"

"That's me," said a tall, black-haired woman who'd gathered with the other nurses for the change-of-shift report.

"Any idea why Mr. W. asked to see a psychiatrist?"

"Nope," she said. Her tone conveyed annoyance at being interrupted from finishing "report" and heading home.

"Was there anything odd about him?" I pressed.

"When I went into the room to check another patient, he asked to see one. That's all I know."

Room 315 was dimly lit. It had gray walls and green and white checkered linoleum-covered floors. A large window at the end of the room looked out to the brick wall on the opposite side of an airshaft. There were four beds in the room—two on each side; all were occupied. The bed in the far left corner of the room had its curtains pulled around it. Loud snoring emanated from behind the fabric.

Mr. W. was in the bed on the right side of the room, closest to the door. His name was printed on a cardboard sign at the foot of the bed. The head of the bed was inclined at a forty-five-degree angle. Mr. W. held an open *New York Post* on his lap.

The other patients were asleep. The man in the next bed lay on his side, snoring lightly, facing away from Mr. W. The faint sound of music came from a transistor radio beneath the sleeping man's pillow.

My psychiatric evaluation would involve a minute dissection of Mr. W.'s presentation—physical, mental, and emotional. Everything would be assessed: whether his fingernails were clipped, his cuticles bitten or ragged, and whether or not he fidgeted, sweated profusely, or showed signs of restlessness or anxiety. I'd assess his demeanor, his verbiage, the emotional tone of his voice, the cadence of speech, his insight, his intellectual capacity, his cognition, and many other things—some quite nuanced. With some patients, it could be a formidable task requiring a careful examination of everything: his thinking, feeling, and behavior—the complete package, its content and presentation.

Standing at the room's entrance, I made my first assessment of Calvin W.

Most post-op patients had a drawn, fatigued look—if only from the aftereffects of anesthesia. But Mr. W. looked well nourished, rested, and robust. He was alert, reading a newspaper. He wore a blue hospital gown. He smelled vaguely of soap, as though he'd recently showered. His skin was the color of light mocha chocolate. He looked to be of medium height and build, was clean-shaven, had a neatly trimmed mustache, and wore wire-rimmed reading glasses, a wedding ring, and a plastic hospital ID band around his left wrist.

Glancing up from the newspaper, he noticed me.

Approaching the bed, I introduced myself.

His eyebrows rose. He dropped the newspaper in his lap and said, "Please, call me Calvin . . . or Cal."

"Sure." I'd long ago abandoned the formality of using patients' last names if they preferred otherwise. Especially in a consultation, it helped form a rapport, a sense of comfort, so the patient might talk openly with a complete stranger who happened to be a psychiatrist.

We shook hands. His grip was firm. His hand was warm and dry. Grunting from some abdominal pain, he straightened himself in the bed. So far nothing was unusual. He seemed normal.

I pulled a nearby chair to the bedside and sat down.

"Cal, I heard you asked to see me."

"Yes, I did," he said. He exhaled audibly, pressed his lips together, and shook his head. Something was amiss.

"What can I do for you?" I asked, intrigued by his request.

His lips curled into a weak smile, but his forehead wrinkled into a burgeoning scowl. He hesitated, as though unsure where to begin. Not an unusual reaction when a complete stranger asks what might be causing some inner turmoil—enough to prompt a request to see a psychiatrist.

"What can you do for me?" he said. "Doc, I don't even know where to begin." He exhaled again very loudly. "It's been only two days, but it feels like I've been here forever."

"What's going on?"

"Lemme give you an example, Doc . . . and it's nothing personal . . ." His voice trailed off. He looked away for a moment and then peered at me as if to gauge my reaction. "I don't wanna offend you."

"Of course not," I said, waiting for some indirect insult.

"I asked to see you at one this afternoon. I asked three different nurses, but it was like talkin' to the walls. And here you are," he said, glancing at his wristwatch, "eleven at night. It took ten hours. That's typical of this place." He shook his head.

This was going to be a tough interview. He had a gripe to get off his chest. I was dealing with a highly disgruntled patient. My legs felt tight.

"I'm sorry it took so long. But I came as soon as I got the call."

It was strange: only one request for a psychiatrist was in the chart. I came to what seemed a logical conclusion about the discrepancy: the nurses were very busy—swamped was more like it—and hadn't gotten around to calling the psychiatry department. After all, Mr. W. hadn't created a disturbance and his request was probably deemed a low-priority issue. And there was nothing about this man that would have alerted the nurses that he was disturbed in some way.

"I don't know how this place keeps going," he continued. "Nobody listens or gives a damn about the patients."

"Uh-huh," I said, nodding my head.

Oh yes, this man is aggrieved.

"Why should it take almost eleven hours to get you over here?"

"I don't know, Mr. W., but—"

"It's Cal, as in Cal Ripken," he said with a chortle.

"I see you're a baseball fan," I said, glancing at the *Post*. It was opened to the sports pages.

"A Yankees fan," he said, nodding.

"They didn't do so great this season," I said, doing my best to deflect his annoyance at the hospital, the personnel, and possibly me. "There's always next year, Cal."

"That's right, Doc." His lips formed the beginnings of a smile.

He seemed to be a regular guy; didn't seem overly resentful of a large hospital's slow-motion machinations—irked, but not unduly so.

I sat at the bedside, trying to figure out what was really bothering Calvin W., otherwise known as Cal—as in Cal Ripken, star shortstop for the Baltimore Orioles at the time.

"I should've asked to see you sooner," he said, "because this place is for the birds."

I wondered if now he would launch into a full-blown tirade about the nurses and doctors conspiring against him, slipping a forbidden substance into his medication, or doing something to him while he was unconscious in the OR.

"Lemme tell you, Doc, the patients don't count around here. Nobody listens, and to tell you the truth, nobody gives a good goddamn."

"How do you mean?"

"From the moment I got here, nobody talked to me. Not the doctors, not the nurses, not the aides . . . nobody. They just handed me this johnny coat, and the doctors came around, put their hands on me, and asked a bunch of questions: 'Does it hurt here? Does it hurt when I do this?' Six or seven come in at a time—and you feel like a guinea pig.

"They talk to each other like you're not even here. They talk about your white counts and your red counts . . . They never ask about my black counts," he added with a chuckle.

I smiled but held back a laugh, not wanting him to think I viewed his troubles as frivolous.

"So they're all standing here, right at my bed, and I gotta lift up my gown and they feel around down there, you know, where the hernia was. They poke and push and ask me to cough while they got a finger poked into my groin, and it's right in front of the women—nurses and the female medical students. It's humiliating.

"Listen, Doc, I know they gotta teach the students, but there's no dignity here. You're just a piece of meat."

"Well, you know, Cal, this is a teaching hospital," I said, aware I sounded defensive.

"But still, patients're human beings, and we oughta be shown some respect. I know how it is because I'm a short-order cook in a busy diner. The place is a damned madhouse, especially at lunchtime. I know how people feel when they're treated like just a number."

He paused. The patient in the next bed coughed and then resumed snoring.

"And I'll tell you another thing," he said, pulling himself up in the bed. "As bad as the doctors are, the nurses are even worse. Of all people, they oughta know better."

"What about the nurses?" I asked, recalling the short shrift I was given at the nursing station.

"One or two of 'em're okay, but most of 'em don't care, and they don't listen. The fact that you're here so many hours after I asked for you is typical. To them, you're just another warm body lyin' in a bed."

I nodded, knowing the hospital could be terribly impersonal. The mammoth size of the place coupled with the huge patient load could make it seem remote and uncaring.

"And if that isn't bad enough, you oughta taste the food," he went on. "Man, I'm a cook, so I know somethin' about food. Damn, it's the worst crap on earth. Okay, so I was on a soft diet this morning . . . *cold* soft-boiled eggs. By the time the food tray gets to you, everythin's cold. The stuff they fed me I wouldn't give to a stray dog."

"I understand, Cal. I eat the hospital food, too."

My thoughts streaked in a diagnostic expedition:

Was Calvin W.'s language coherent, spoken in an orderly way, or did he speak in a manner typical of schizophrenia? His words were connected logically, coherently, and sequentially. His speech wasn't pressured or expansive; it was straight, direct—and there was no evidence of disordered thinking. *Scratch out schizophrenia.*

Was he unduly suspicious or guarded? Not remotely. He was dissatisfied, but not delusional. He was open and cordial, wanted to be called by his first name, and seemed comfortable with me. *Eliminate paranoia.*

Was he aggrieved? Sure, but in a hospital like Manhattan, who wouldn't be?

"And another thing, Doc," he continued. "These hospital gowns're humiliating. This afternoon I had to use the bathroom. And you know . . . these stupid things tie in the back with this dumb string, and you're exposed. And there I am, makin' my way to the toilet, my ass hangin' out, when some lady comes to visit the guy in the next bed. I tried to cover up, but it was too late. So she just turns away, pretends she doesn't see my behind. I was so damned embarrassed. My ass was hanging out like a hunka brown meat."

He snickered and then began laughing.

I realized a grin had broken out on my face.

"I understand completely," I said. "Is anything else bothering you, Cal?"

"Ah, just the usual hospital crap. This poor guy over here," he said, jabbing a thumb toward the snoring patient in the next bed. "They check on him every hour, so I can't get any asleep. Who can sleep with three other guys in a room, snorin' and spittin' up, coughin' and passin' gas? I just wanna get outta here."

There wasn't a single thing he said that wasn't true. Manhattan Hospital was a huge medical assembly line. A guy like Calvin W. could feel lost in a sea of indifference—simply passing through the place with monitors beeping, IVs dripping, portable X-ray and EKG machines being wheeled into rooms at all hours, nurses scurrying, porters mopping, aides changing bed linens, medical students and attending physicians making rounds, interns and residents popping in and out—it was a conveyor belt with little or no time for compassionate care or the ordinary niceties of life.

Calvin W.'s feelings were right on the money—expectable and fully appropriate in these circumstances.

I'd already arrived at a simple conclusion: despite his unhappiness with the hospital's undeniable indifference and the impersonal atmosphere of it all, there was absolutely nothing wrong psychiatrically with Calvin W. He was perfectly sane.

He was simply a dissatisfied patient—a customer with complaints—but an in-touch, sensible, and likable guy.

He took me in with eyebrows raised. I had the distinct feeling he wanted me to make excuses for his unpleasant experience. Was I going to explain how the staff was overworked and underpaid, that new patients flooded the place every hour, that working conditions weren't great? Would I be an apologist for the hospital?

I leaned forward and said, "Cal, I don't understand something."

"What's that, Doc?"

"Why'd you call me?"

"Why'd I call you?" His eyes widened in disbelief. "I just told you . . ."

"I don't understand." This was truly befuddling. A thousand thoughts streaked through my mind.

"What don't you understand?" he said, an edge of annoyance creeping into his voice.

I hesitated and then came out with it. "Well, as a psychiatrist, I'm not sure—"

"*What?*"

"I don't know why you asked to see a psychiatrist."

"A psychiatrist? You're a *psychiatrist*?"

"Yes."

"A head shrinker? You mean I'm talkin' to a *shrink*?"

"Yes. You asked to see a psychiatrist."

His mouth opened, or more aptly, his jaw dropped. Nearly to the floor. And his eyes looked like bulging globes in their sockets. The whites showed above his brown irises. He sat there in wide-eyed astonishment. His chin trembled.

Heat spread through my face. Here I was, sitting at the bedside of a completely sane man who'd asked to see a psychiatrist. And yet he was amazed—completely shocked—when I told him my specialty. What on earth was going on?

Suddenly, his head reared back, his mouth opened, his eyes closed, and he laughed. It was a hearty sound, deep, resonant, and genuine. He couldn't stop laughing. Both hands slipped onto his lower abdomen; he held his belly as his body shook with laughter.

Had I hallucinated being told he wanted to see a psychiatrist?

Not a chance. I'd seen the entry in Calvin W.'s chart.

Was this some ill-conceived joke?

Calvin W. finally stopped laughing. A smile lingered on his lips. He shook his head from side to side. "It's unbelievable," he said, chortling. "This is exactly what I'm talkin' about. *Exactly*." He slapped his palm on the bedsheet.

"You mean you *didn't* ask to see a psychiatrist?"

"You know what, Doc? Like I said, after lunch I asked to see the head doctor," he said, stifling a laugh. "I told the nurse I wanted to see the head *doctor*—the chief, the boss, the guy in charge of things. Not a *head* doctor."

"You mean an administrator?"

He nodded, closing his eyes as his hand covered his mouth.

I felt a smile spread over my face. I tried to suffocate a laugh, but a snort bubbled up from my throat and then erupted in a riptide of laugher.

When Calvin W. heard my guffaws, he began laughing again.

Soon we were both nearly convulsing with laughter.

"Oh, Doc, I shouldn't laugh this way," he said, holding his abdomen. "It hurts my belly. But I can't help it. It's so funny, it's pathetic. Here I am, asking for the head *doctor*, the head of the department, and they send me a *head* doctor, a *shrink*. It's amazing."

Now it made perfect sense: here I was wearing a jacket and tie—not hospital whites like the interns and residents, and not donned in the white lab coat worn by attending surgeons. And Calvin W. assumed—reasonably—I was an administrator. He thought I was the head physician—the guy to whom he could lodge his complaints.

Not only did it take ten hours for me to arrive, but I was the wrong guy—a *head* doctor.

Our laughter dampened down to a few snickers.

"You know," he said, looking directly into my eyes, "you're the first doctor who sat down and talked to me. A *shrink*."

"That's what we do, Cal. We talk with people."

"Yeah, well, you're the first one who listened to my bitchin'."

I nodded, realizing our talk—our so-called psychiatric interview—was over. Though he hadn't asked for a shrink, Calvin W. had finally spoken with someone who listened. He'd griped and groused; he had gotten some grievances off his chest.

And he probably felt much better. Now he'd have something funny to tell his wife and kids when he got home.

I didn't quite know why, but for some reason I felt I hadn't wasted my time. It seemed I'd served a useful purpose talking with him, and I had the strangest feeling—it was something intuitive—perhaps Calvin W. had something more to discuss.

After a momentary pause, he leaned toward me and asked, "Hey, you're a doctor, right? An MD?"

"Yes."

"I mean, you went to medical school and learned all that good stuff—medicine and surgery, right?"

"Yes, I did."

"And then you got to be a shrink?"

"Sure."

"I hope you don't mind my sayin' 'shrink.'"

"Nah. I hear it all the time."

He pursed his lips.

I sensed he was taking my temperature about something—and it was important to him.

He waited for a few moments, looking like he was going to speak, but said nothing. Then he sighed and finally began. "Maybe you can clear somethin' up for me." His voice lowered. He was no longer smiling. For the first time, his eyes darted away.

"I can try."

He nodded, as though he'd decided to say something.

"I had this operation, you know, this hernia thing?"

"Yeah?"

"Well," he said haltingly, "I'm not sure what they did to me."

"You mean the surgery? What was involved?"

"You got it. What the hell'd they do down there?" His right index finger pointed to his groin.

"Well, Cal, they fixed the hernia."

"But I don't understand what they did to me."

"Didn't the doctors explain the surgery?"

"Nope. They didn't say a damned thing. They just felt around, stuck their fingers down there, and asked me to cough. Then they knocked me out and did the operation."

"Cal, do you know what a hernia is?"

"It's like some kinda rupture, right? Somethin' inside me ruptured?"

"No. Not at all," I said, realizing the guy didn't have a clue about what was done to or for him.

"A hernia means that one part of your insides has slipped from an area where it belongs and slid over to where it doesn't. In your case a part of your large intestine—you know what that is, right?"

"It's my gut. After the stomach comes the intestine, right?"

"Right. Well, a hernia means that part of your body wall got weakened," I said, pointing to my own lower abdomen. "And your intestine began sliding to where it doesn't belong." My hand moved down toward my groin.

I paused, trying to think of an analogy. It suddenly came to me.

"You a football fan?" I asked.

"Oh yeah. The Giants," he said as his eyes brightened.

We were getting to familiar territory.

"Then you know what encroachment is, right?"

"I sure do."

"Well, your gut began to encroach into an area where it didn't belong. It began sliding down this narrow canal—it's called the inguinal canal—and it slid farther down over the last few years. The danger was this little bit of intestine could get squeezed and twisted in this narrow space, and its blood supply could get cut off.

"So the surgeon went into that little canal, pushed the gut back into the belly area, where it belongs, and then sewed up your body wall. No more encroachment."

"Uh-huh. I get it. So the gut's gonna stay where it belongs."

"That's right."

"So how come whenever they examined me they stuck their finger down there and asked me to cough?"

"You mean they slid a finger up beside your balls, right?"

"You got it. Right into my balls."

"Well, this narrow canal leads down to the scrotum, the sac that holds your balls. So they stick a finger down there to see how far down the intestine may've slipped. If enough time passed, the gut would eventually start encroaching into your scrotum. But your gut never got that far."

"But this hernia and this operation . . . Did it affect me down there . . . my balls?" His eyes shifted away from me.

"No, Cal. It had nothing to do with your balls. Not a damned thing."

His eyes met mine. "But the spot where they cut me open, it's right near them. It's right by my groin."

"I know. That's where they went in and pushed the gut back where it belongs. And they sewed it back into your belly. But it has nothing to do with your balls . . . or with your sex life."

"But there're nerves down there."

"This had nothing to do with the nerves. Nothing was touched."

"You're sure?"

"I'm absolutely sure. Let me tell you something," I said as his eyes locked onto mine. "I've never heard of a hernia repair where it affected a man's sex life. It just doesn't happen. *Ever.*"

His lips spread into a smile. "Hey, that's good to hear. Because I gotta tell you, my wife and I have always had a good life together, if you know what I mean."

"Of course I do. But let me assure you, Cal, you'll be able to perform just fine. It'll be the same as always."

His face slackened with relief. He nodded and leaned back on his pillow. He closed his eyes and exhaled through pursed lips. Then a sly smile began forming on his lips and his eyes grew brighter. The change was evident, even in the room's dim light.

The ward was very quiet, except for the faint ribbon of sound from the other guy's radio.

"That's the best news I've heard since I've been here," he said. "Thanks, Doc."

"No sweat, Cal. It's been a pleasure talking with you." I stood and moved the chair back to a corner.

Grimacing from the surgical wound, he leaned toward me with his hand extended. We shook hands.

"You'll be going home tomorrow," I said. "In a week or so, the pain will be gone. And you'll be able to resume your normal activities. *All* of them."

We held eye contact for another moment.

He nodded.

I returned the nod.

"Well, I gotta go," I said.

"Sure. You got other patients to see, right?"

"Right." I turned and began walking toward the door.

"Hey, Doc," he called in a half whisper.

I turned back toward him.

"Thanks for takin' the time to explain things. I appreciate it."

I nodded again.

"I'm glad you came to see me."

"I'm glad, too. I enjoyed talking with you." I felt a smile come over my face.

"You set me straight, Doc."

"Well," I said, "I'm the *head* doctor . . ."

We laughed softly.

We waved to each other as I approached the door.

"Stay well," I said.

"You too, Doc."

I turned and headed down the corridor. I realized I felt very good—even elated.

I'd actually accomplished something, helped a patient negotiate his way through a personal minicrisis of sorts.

At the nursing station, the nurses had finished giving report. Ms. Lowry was gone, but her replacement, Ms. Edwards asked, "How's Mr. W.?"

"Oh, he's fine."

"What's his problem?"

"Oh . . . just some personal issues he wanted to talk about. No big deal."

"You gonna make an entry in his chart?" she asked.

"Sure," I said, going to the chart rack. I pulled the metal-bound record from its slot and sat on a rolling secretarial chair.

I decided the only entry I'd make was that Mr. W. and I talked about some personal matters.

Yes, he'd gotten some things off his chest.

And then we talked about some very personal concerns.

Afterword

Some might interpret Calvin W.'s request to see the head doctor as an unconscious wish to talk to a psychiatrist about his deepest concern—the effect of the hernia operation on his sexual functioning.

Others might argue such an interpretation is far too Freudian and a real stretch.

But no matter how you view his request, one thing is abundantly clear: Calvin W. knew next to nothing about his physical condition and the surgical procedure to remedy it. For all he knew, the nerves to his genitals were severed, and he would never again function sexually. On a very deep level, he was terrified that an important element of his life was compromised, if not completely gone. When he was given the opportunity to talk to me, maybe more so because I was a shrink in addition to being a physician, Calvin W.'s fears emerged.

The consultation's big "takeaway" for me was the importance of doctors talking with their patients. Throughout my career, I've encountered many patients who, despite being in prolonged treatment, were misinformed or ignorant about their medical conditions. Physicians in all specialties frequently neglect to fully discuss with patients their diagnoses and treatment plans. The end result: patients are burdened with frightening and unrealistic fantasies.

More than ever before, physician-patient communication suffers in today's medical environment. Corporate-based group practices require doctors to maximize the number of patients seen each day to offset reimbursement cutbacks from insurers. In addition, practices must hire additional professionals to process the reams of insurance and government forms presented in their offices. These factors create financial pressures for doctors to see as many patients as possible. Physicians typically allot approximately fifteen minutes for a patient visit, scarcely enough time for an examination, let alone for a full-fledged consultation.

Nowadays, in many places, even though you may have a family practitioner, if you're admitted to the hospital, you're assigned a *hospitalist*, a physician employed by the hospital who knows little or nothing about you, other than what the electronic medical records on file reveal. At the time you and your family are most in need of the support and guidance a family doctor can provide, a vital connection is ruptured.

Long gone is the family doctor who made house calls. My father was a physician in the days when house calls were routine. He knew each of his patients, many of whom had been with him for decades. He went to their homes when they were too sick to come to his office, knew their children, and spent time with the family as needed. The comfort level between my father and his patients was such that questions were asked and information flowed freely. A trusting relationship was formed and nourished over the years.

Today, if you're affluent and want the kind of attention all patients once enjoyed, you can find a physician who has established a concierge practice. For an annual fee, this doctor will spend the time and provide the personalized service once afforded all patients in the days of the house call. But there are very few concierge practices, and becoming a patient in one of them can be an expensive proposition. And even in these practices, if you're admitted to a hospital, you're assigned a hospitalist during your stay.

Over the last decade or two the interface between patients and their doctors has changed radically.

Poor communication now occurs even in *psychiatry*, the sole specialty that has traditionally placed a premium on talking with and listening to patients. Many psychiatrists now work in multidisciplinary groups. Others conduct *medication* practices—which are becoming more common—spending ten minutes with each patient every few months for medication checks. Whereas psychiatrists formerly saw eight or nine patients each day for forty-five-minute sessions, many now see thirty to forty patients in a single day. Psychotherapy is relegated to other professionals—psychologists and social workers, if it's done at all.

Frequently, no psychotherapy is available to chronically mentally ill patients.[2]

And how does this all relate to Calvin W.?

When you reflect back on his story, you see it was all about poor communication. From the time his hernia was first diagnosed, before he ever set foot into the hospital, until the moment at his bedside when we discussed his surgery and manhood, the medical profession failed him in one very important way: no one took the time to talk with and listen to him.

Regrettably, there are many more people like Calvin W., worrying needlessly, because the medical profession is ill—suffering from the chronic condition of poor communication.

---

2. Over the years, studies have shown that severely ill patients (those with chronic schizophrenia, bipolar disorder, or recurrent major depression) do much better when treated with a combination of medication and psychotherapy than if treated with either modality, alone. Bruce E. Wexler and Domenic V. Cicchetti, "The Outpatient Treatment of Depression: Implications of Outcome Research for Clinical Practice," *Journal of Nervous and Mental Disease* 180, no. 5 (1992): 277–86.

Baptism by Fire

When she was brought to Manhattan Hospital's psychiatric emergency room, Patricia A.'s agony was unmistakable.

She was a gaunt-looking thirty-five-year-old woman who paced back and forth, muttering feverishly and wringing her hands. Dark circles crouched beneath her red-rimmed eyes. When she turned to her mother to speak, her words were barely coherent.

I was working in the emergency room that evening as part of my first-year residency rotation. My daytime duties involved working on the third-floor women's ward.

Noting Patricia's condition, I wanted to get history from her mother without Patricia being present; but fearing she might wander off, I asked a security guard to watch her. Patricia remained in the reception area while I interviewed her mother, Rose, in my office.

"Patricia's a complete wreck," Rose said, stifling a sob. "Her husband, Leonard, died of a heart attack three months ago. My God, he was only forty years old. He went to the gym that morning. Then, while he was in the shower, he just . . . he just dropped dead." From Rose's description, Leonard was the victim of sudden cardiac death—his heart began beating erratically, virtually quivering, and failed to pump blood. It was an unexpected and tragic end to a seemingly healthy young man.

"But that's not the whole story," Rose continued. "Yes, Patricia was shocked when Leonard died. It was a terrible blow . . . and so unexpected. I also felt my world had collapsed; after all, he was like a son to me. But Patricia was always a strong woman, and it seemed she would deal with the loss . . . at first.

"The terrible thing—on top of his dying—was what happened at the funeral home," Rose said, doing her best to stifle her tears. "Although she asked for a closed casket, Patricia wanted one last look at Leonard before we left for the cemetery. The funeral director tried to talk her out of it, but she insisted. That's when it happened." Rose swallowed hard. Her hands began trembling. "What she saw was horrible. You see, Doctor, Leonard was a very tall man—he was six five—and when the people at the funeral home set him in the coffin, he didn't fit."

Rose could no longer hold back her emotions. Her shoulders shook and tears cascaded from her eyes. "When Patricia looked at Leonard, she saw that to get him into the casket, they broke his neck. His head was twisted to the side . . . and . . . and . . . it was jammed into a corner of the coffin."

I tried imagining a bereaved widow looking into a casket, seeing her husband's neck snapped and his head angled obscenely into the coffin's corner. My guts nearly recoiled at the image.

Giving Rose a few minutes to compose herself, I walked to the waiting room and asked Patricia to accompany me to the consultation room.

She stared ahead. Her eyes appeared unfocused.

"Can you talk with me?"

"I . . . I . . . I . . ." Glottal sounds erupted from her throat, nothing more.

Was she catatonic?

Clearly, Patricia was incapable of participating in any discussion; and it could be injurious for her to hear her mother's emotion-filled description of what happened at the funeral parlor. I signaled to a security guard to continue watching Patricia closely.

Back in the consultation room, I explained to Rose I thought it better that our conversation continued without her daughter and assured her Patricia was being watched.

"Patricia doesn't sleep or eat," Rose said. "She's lost more than ten pounds. She stopped working. She paces all day. And she talks to herself; she just keeps saying, 'Leonard . . . Leonard . . . ' She told me about a dream she has over and over, of Leonard hanging from a tree. His neck looks like it did in the coffin."

"So, the dream reenacts what happened at the funeral home?"

"Yes. And right after the funeral she keeps thinking she sees Leonard's body in that coffin. It's like a vision of some kind. Don't you call them flashbacks, Doctor?"

"Yes, that's what they're called."

"This is more than ordinary mourning, isn't it?"

"Yes. Patricia's developed a serious illness on top of her grief."

"She's very depressed, isn't she?" Rose asked.

"Yes. It sounds like post-traumatic stress disorder, with severe depression, along with her grief."

"But what worries me most is what happened yesterday."

"What's that?"

"She was mumbling. I couldn't understand most of it, but she was talking to Leonard. I think she's hearing his voice. And I heard her say she'd see him soon."

"Meaning she's thinking of killing herself, that she'll join him?"

"Yes," Rose whispered, sobbing into her hands.

"Has she tried to hurt herself?"

"Not so far. She's been living with me since Leonard died. But I can't watch her twenty-four hours a day. I think she needs to be hospitalized. That's why I brought her here."

"You did the right thing. We'll admit her and get her stabilized.

Right now she needs to be protected."

As the paperwork was completed, Patricia remained mute, staring into space. It was impossible to know if she understood, or even cared about what was happening.

"I hate to think of her in the hospital," Rose said, dabbing her eyes with a tissue. "She'll be on a locked ward with very disturbed people, won't she, Doctor?"

"Everyone goes to a locked ward first. My guess is in a few weeks, she'll be well enough to go to the community ward, which isn't locked. But first we have to get her out of this state."[3]

Ten days later I met with Dr. Jamison—my supervising psychiatrist—in his office near the ward's dayroom.

"I'm very worried," he said. "Patricia A. has petitioned for discharge."

"I've seen her every day," I said. "She's improved on the medication but still seems to be a suicide risk."

"Yes. There's a certain tranquillity about her that's disturbing. It's a sense of resignation you see when someone's decided to end her life. I think she's made peace with a terrible decision."

"To join her husband."

"It's a reunion fantasy," Jamison said, leaning back in his chair. "And the liaison attorney has put the papers in for a hearing. It's set for Monday morning."

"She has an attorney?"

"Yes," Jamison said. "His name's James Greenwood. He's in private practice and does this additional work for the state. Patricia asked to see him, which is a bit unusual."

---

3. The New York State Mental Hygiene Law (Section 9.39) states a patient may be involuntarily hospitalized in a psychiatric facility if there is reasonable cause to believe the person has a mental illness for which immediate observation, care, and treatment in a hospital is appropriate and which is likely to result in serious harm to him/herself or others.

"How so?"

"Usually Greenwood makes rounds and asks patients on the wards if they want to be discharged. If they do, a hearing is mandatory. But Patricia *asked* to see him. That's how intent she is on getting out of here and ending her life."

"So, you'll testify?" I asked.

"Ordinarily, I would, but I'll be away. I have a conference in Chicago."

"Why not postpone the hearing?"

"I can't," Jamison said. "New York's Mental Hygiene Law requires us to respect the patient's civil rights. It's written in stone. When an involuntarily hospitalized patient requests a hearing, the demand—and that's what it is, a *demand*—must be met expeditiously. *Expeditiously* has been interpreted as meaning within one week of the request. The judge comes for hearings on Mondays *only*. If we postpone the hearing, the delay means we'll be violating her civil rights; there could be severe legal repercussions for the hospital and for me, personally."

Jamison paused. "So, the alternative is simple: you'll testify."

Voltage shot through me.

As a first-year resident, I had limited experience, and it was zero when it came to a legal contest over a patient's civil liberties. Ordinarily, the attending psychiatrist testified, justifying the hospital's refusal to discharge a patient because she was mentally ill and likely dangerous, either to herself or to others. Though I'd sat in on a few hearings, I'd never defended the decision to keep an unwilling patient on the hospital's locked ward. Usually a hearing was a legal tug-of-war.

It would be my initiation into the law's interface with medicine and psychiatry.

It could be my baptism by fire.

It was nine o'clock on a clear Monday morning.

The ward dayroom was set up for the hearing. The couches and chairs had been pushed to one side of the expanse. A six-foot-long oak table stood at the end of the room. An American flag stood on a stanchion at one end of the table, and the New York State flag stood at the opposite side. The dayroom had been transformed into a makeshift courtroom.

Judge Hobbs sat behind the table. He was an overweight man wearing a dark suit—no black robes. He had a kindly looking face made more so by the wire-rimmed glasses perched on his nose. The court stenographer sat beside him.

I sat at the far end of a table set perpendicular to the one behind which the judge presided. The tables formed a large T.

Jorge Sanchez, the hospital's attorney, took the seat to my left.

Patricia A.'s advocate, James Greenwood, sat at the same table, but to my right. A squat, thick-necked man with a severe under-bite, Greenwood looked like a surly bulldog.

To say I was nervous would be a gross understatement. My heartbeat drubbed in my wrists and my underarms were wet.

Patricia A. sat to Greenwood's right, nearest the judge. She appeared far more composed than when I'd first seen her but still seemed remote, as though some remnant of catatonic paralysis simmered within her. The notion of discussing her as though she weren't even present was unsettling. It seemed bizarre, completely antithetical to the very underpinnings of the doctor-patient relationship.

But this was commonplace in the forensic setting.

Before the hearing I'd met briefly with Sanchez to go over my testimony. He told me a little about James Greenwood. "He's an aggressive stickler for civil rights," Sanchez began. "His position is simple: he thinks patients' rights are consistently violated by the hospital. At heart he's a libertarian. And he hates psychiatry. He thinks it's a bogus specialty. For him it's all about individual freedom and civil rights, not about making medical decisions for impaired people."

Just recalling Sanchez's words filled me with dread. It would be a grueling morning.

"As far as your testimony is concerned," Sanchez had said, "I'll ask you to describe Mrs. A.'s condition. Just tell it like it is. The facts will speak for themselves."

Sanchez and Greenwood recited the issues of the case. Though they weren't physicians, they were meticulously thorough, and it was obvious they knew plenty of medical terminology. The stenographer's fingers flew over her little machine, recording every word.

The judge listened, occasionally jotting notes.

After the attorneys had presented their cases, the judge turned to me. He asked me to state my name and position at the hospital. He then asked me to raise my right hand—no Bible.

With my hand raised, I swore to tell the truth.

Sanchez took me through direct examination. He asked me to describe the emergency-room evaluation of Patricia. Step-by-step Sanchez had me explain Patricia's reaction to her husband's sudden death and of seeing his mangled corpse at the funeral home.

I described her initial presentation, the interview with her mother, Patricia's sleeplessness and nightmares, the daytime flashbacks, and her increasing isolation and debilitating depression, along with her inability to work. I also detailed her virtually catatonic state when she came to the hospital, aware Patricia sat nearby, hearing every word. I tried dealing with her presence by forcing myself to pretend she wasn't there.

Sanchez then asked me to describe bereavement as a normal and expectable occurrence after the death of a loved one and had me contrast that to Patricia's reaction.

"So then, you're saying, Doctor, that Mrs. A.'s presentation involves a complicated form of bereavement?"

"Yes."

"Please tell Judge Hobbs about the complications in her clinical presentation," Sanchez continued.

He had me focus on Patricia's conversations with her dead husband. Sanchez asked about the implications of these auditory hallucinations and what they might portend. I emphasized the likelihood of suicide, given Patricia's mental and emotional states, including not only depression, but post-traumatic stress disorder—all superimposed on the grieving process.

Greenwood scribbled furiously on a legal pad during the direct examination. I found this disconcerting, knowing he was busily refining his cross-examination questions. I did my best to ignore him but felt certain he'd come at me with bared fangs.

"Doctor," Sanchez said, "what caused Mrs. A. to develop post-traumatic stress disorder in addition to her depression and bereavement?"

"It was the sight of her husband's mutilated body."

"Could you please tell the judge exactly what post-traumatic stress disorder is?"

I didn't want to sound textbookish, but it was important to describe the condition. "Post-traumatic stress disorder is caused by witnessing a horrific sight, something beyond the range of ordinary human circumstances," I explained. "It can involve violence or a terrifying situation where a person's life is threatened, or witnessing a violent death or the aftermath of violence or a death. Mrs. A.'s seeing her husband's broken neck caused the disorder."

"How did it do that?" Sanchez asked.

"She was psychologically assaulted by the sight."

Knowing my words could have a sledgehammer impact on Mrs. A., I avoided looking in her direction. Patricia remained a blurred presence off to my right.

"Seeing her husband's broken neck made her recoil in horror. She couldn't get it out of her thoughts."

Greenwood continued scribbling.

"And why was Patricia A. hospitalized?" Sanchez asked.

"Because she was so deeply affected, she couldn't function. She developed an agitated depression, and her mother believes—as do I—she's most likely suicidal. She was talking to the imaginary voice of her dead husband and said she would see him soon. In other words, she's been experiencing auditory hallucinations, hearing her husband's voice and answering him as though he's present. She has to be protected from her wish to join him in death."

Dense silence descended on the dayroom after Sanchez finished the direct examination. The court reporter asked for a break to refill her machine with a new roll of paper.

I waited, anticipating a blistering string of questions from Greenwood. My mouth felt parched. I sipped some water. My lower left eyelid quivered—blepharospasm—a surefire sign of nervousness.

The court reporter nodded to the judge.

"Cross-examination," said the judge.

Greenwood stared at me. His eyes smoldered with hostility.

My heart thrashed in my chest.

"Correct me if I'm wrong, Doctor," Greenwood said, "but didn't you say a minute ago that it's *likely* that Patricia became suicidal?"

"Yes." Wariness flooded me. My toes curled. My voice sounded scratchy. I hoped it wouldn't warble. My lower left eyelid kept quivering.

"What do you mean by *likely*?"

"That she's probably suicidal."

"Probably? What do you mean by 'probably'?"

"It's more likely to happen than not."

"Fine, Doctor," Greenwood said. His eyes bored into me.

I didn't know why, but I felt I'd somehow made a major concession.

"Your use of the word *probably* is crucial here. Just so you know, in the law, when we talk about probability, we're talking about something being fifty-one percent or more likely to happen. Do you understand that?"

"Yes."

Pure condescension. Overbearing and obnoxious.

"So if something's fifty-one percent likely to occur, that leaves a forty-nine percent chance it will *not* occur, right?"

"Objection," Sanchez called. "Mr. Greenwood knows it's a sliding scale. Something can be probable because there's a fifty-one percent or *greater* chance it'll happen. For all we know, there's a ninety-five percent chance the patient is suicidal."

"Sustained," ruled the judge.

"Your Honor," Greenwood said, turning to the judge. "Mr. Sanchez just answered for the doctor. He's coaching the witness."

"The objection is still sustained, Mr. Greenwood."

"Your Honor, I'm sure you noticed Mr. Sanchez said, 'For all we know.' My point in raising this question is the doctor's talking about *probability*. The fact of the matter is simple: there's no accurate measure of the patient's so-called suicidality. It's nothing more than guesswork."

"So noted, Mr. Greenwood," said the judge. "The doctor's obviously making a judgment call based on the factors he enumerated on direct examination."

Greenwood flipped a page on his legal pad and turned to me. "Doctor, isn't it true that of all medical specialties psychiatry's the least scientific?"

"No. That's a common misconception," I said. "There've been enormous advances in understanding the biochemistry of mental illness. In fact, the latest medications have had an enormous impact on—"

"But, Doctor, isn't it true that you—"

"*Objection*," Sanchez shot. "Mr. Greenwood's interrupting the witness. He didn't finish his answer."

"Mr. Greenwood, don't interrupt," warned the judge. "Let the witness complete his answer." Turning to me, he said, "Doctor, are you finished with your answer?"

I did my best to recover my train of thought. "I was just going to say the latest psychiatric medications have changed the landscape of psychiatry as a medical specialty. We're much better able to control symptoms."

"Control *symptoms*?" Greenwood asked as his eyebrows rose toward his hairline. "Don't you mean by altering the patient's brain chemistry?"

"Yes."

"The medication does that, correct?"

"Yes."

"So psychiatrists engage in a form of mind control by altering people's brain chemistry, don't they?"

"Call it whatever you want, Mr. Greenwood. All physicians prescribe medications that alter the body's chemistry."

"How do you decide what medication you're going to use to alter someone's brain chemistry?"

"You decide empirically by using what you know based on your training, education, and experience. And you use the patient's presentation and history as guidelines."

"Speaking of history, Doctor, isn't it true that you depend on what a patient tells you to make a diagnosis?"

"Not exclusively. We evaluate the patient's circumstances and psychiatric presentation in addition to the history."

I did my best not to sound didactic, to avoid a pedantic lecture since Greenwood was being incredibly disingenuous. But something was clear: it would be push-pull, veer left, shift right. My every utterance would be subjected to Greenwood's agenda-driven dissection. He'd play word games and resort to a microexamination of anything I said in the service of his intention—to get Patricia A. released from the hospital.

My heart drubbed a tattoo in my chest. Even my fingertips seemed to pulse.

"Tell me, Doctor," Greenwood went on, "psychiatrists depend on history, don't they?"

"Physicians in every specialty depend on patients' histories, along with objective findings," I countered. "History taking isn't unique to psychiatry."

"But you depend on a history of symptoms, don't you? Psychiatry comes up short on actual *signs* of illness, doesn't it?"

"That's not true. A *symptom* is a subjective complaint—like pain or nausea. In psychiatry, a *symptom* can be feeling sad or experiencing hopelessness. In medicine, a *sign* of illness is *objective*, something you can actually see or hear . . . like a fever, a heart murmur, or a swollen liver.

"In psychiatry, a *sign* could be a patient crying, sweating excessively, or someone who's disheveled. Or it could be severe agitation and pacing, or someone who's delusional and claims to be God. Those are *signs* of mental illness."

"But, Doctor, isn't there a great deal of debate within the field of psychiatry about diagnostic categories?"

"Yes, there's debate about classifying and coding some mental disorders. That doesn't invalidate a thorough evaluation of someone. In fact, the technical diagnosis may sometimes be secondary to what's really important—whether or not the patient's lost touch with reality. And if the patient *is* psychotic, the burning issue is whether or not the psychosis makes her dangerous to herself or others. That's what counts when deciding whether or not to admit someone to the hospital."

"Lost touch with reality?" Greenwood asked. His eyebrows rose again. "Exactly who defines reality, Doctor? You? The hospital?

Other doctors? A textbook? Some manual? What and who defines reality?"

"I can only say reality is defined by common agreement. It's defined by consensual understanding of the world."

"What does 'consensual understanding' mean?" Greenwood shook his head in feigned befuddlement. His lips formed the beginnings of a smirk.

"It means we all agree on a certain reality in the world. I can only explain it by example."

"Oh, please, Doctor, go ahead."

That smirk had yet to fully appear on his face, but it was clearly present in his voice. The guy was being irritatingly smug. My legs felt so tight I thought they might seize into a contraction.

"Right now six of us are sitting in this dayroom," I said. "If one of us sees a face on the wall and the other five don't, then the person seeing the face is experiencing a visual hallucination. That person is out of touch with the consensual reality, with the mutually agreed upon world as it exists."

"So, Doctor, if I see a face on that wall over there," Greenwood rejoined, pointing to the far wall, "that gives you the right to hospitalize me against my will?"

"If that face is talking and telling you to kill yourself or to kill other people, then yes. The hospital—really, the community—has the right to extrude you and put you where you won't hurt yourself or anyone else. A place where you can be protected from yourself and where other people can be protected from you. A place where you can be treated until your ability to deal realistically with the world is restored."

"How can you know I'm going to hurt myself or other people?"

"A patient comes to the hospital and a history comes along, too. If there's a history of violent behavior, or suicidal thinking, or an attempt at suicide, then it's pretty clear: either the patient has to be protected or both the patient and other people need protection."

"Doctor, isn't it true there are no biological markers in any mental illness, other than in something like Alzheimer's? There are no physical findings in any of the other mental illnesses indicating pathology, correct?"

"None have been definitely defined or described at this time."[4]

"Then how can you consider depression a true illness, since it lacks any biological markers or organic findings?"

"I think it's ridiculous to say depression isn't a legitimate illness that needs treatment just because our biological knowledge is incomplete at this time. Markers will probably be found in the future."

"But, Doctor," Greenwood pushed on, "feelings of depression can occur in many situations, not just depressive illness, if you want to call it that. It can even be a *normal* response to bad things happening. How can you consider it pathologic?"

"If you want to think that way, Mr. Greenwood, then you can't consider hypertension pathologic, since it happens in many different situations. And it's a normal physiologic response to stress. By your line of reasoning, hypertension shouldn't be considered *real* or *legitimate*, and we shouldn't treat it. We should just let patients continue on and eventually have a stroke."

"But we can measure hypertension, can't we?" he said.

"And we can see depression when it happens."

Greenwood blinked a couple of times, looked down at his legal pad and then at me, and said, "Are you aware that some psychiatrists—I'm thinking about Dr. Thomas Szasz, a noted psychiatrist and analyst—believe the psychiatric establishment makes negative judgments about people whose behavior they find disturbing and about which they disapprove; so they view them as being sick?"

"That's not the thinking of mainstream psychiatry."

---

4. This hearing occurred before the latest biological markers and biochemical abnormalities for certain mental illnesses were discovered.

"You *do* make judgments about people's behavior, don't you?"

"Yes, I do."

"And you concede you're making a judgment about Patricia A., don't you?"

"Yes. It's part of my job."

"Now, Doctor, on direct examination you said that mourning, or bereavement, follows the death or loss of a loved one, correct?"

"Yes."

"So it's expectable that someone would mourn after the death of a husband?"

"Yes, of course."

"And, Doctor, do you acknowledge that bereavement has certain stages?"

"Yes, that's generally accepted."

"And what stage of bereavement is Patricia in right now?"

"It's impossible to define a specific stage of her bereavement right now. I have no doubt she's angry and depressed, but it's not *just* simple grief. Her reaction is complicated by post-traumatic stress disorder and by profound depression. It's a clouded picture."

"If it's clouded, then how can you be so certain about what's going on?"

"I have to look at the entire picture, the whole landscape."

Despite my best efforts to the contrary, I was sure I sounded how I felt—very wary, even hypervigilant. Answering Greenwood's questions was the verbal equivalent of walking barefoot on shards of glass. He was doing his best to snare me into tangential cul-de-sacs and minor fine points, even irrelevancies. He was attempting to point out minute distinctions that made no difference in the long run. He'd do his best to obscure the danger of leaving Patricia's severe depression and PTSD untreated.

Greenwood continued. "So, since Mrs. A. lost her husband in this traumatic way, you would expect her to be in an acute state of shock and to be bereaved, correct?"

"Yes, that's expectable."

"And that occurred, correct?"

"Yes."

"Now, Doctor, do bereaved people ever dream about the deceased person?"

"Yes, they can."

"Repeatedly?"

"Yes, that can happen."

"If someone loses a loved one in the horrible fashion Mrs. A. did—a sudden death in a shower stall—can those dreams be so intense they wake her up at night?"

"It can happen, yes."

"And tell me this, Doctor . . ." Greenwood went on, barely missing a beat. "Do bereaved people think about the deceased during the day and at night?"

"Yes, they often do."

"Especially for the first few months after a sudden traumatic death?"

"Yes."

"Do bereaved people cry when thinking about their lost loved ones?"

"Yes, they do."

"And that's especially true if the death was traumatic and unexpected, such as dropping dead in a shower stall?"

"Yes, that's certainly possible."

"And isn't it true that recently bereaved people often think they see the deceased person in public places?"

"Yes, they sometimes have an illusion like that—a misperception—misinterpreting something they see. It's really a wish to see the loved one again."

"And you've already conceded that Mr. A.'s death was traumatic for Mrs. A., yes?"

"Yes."

"So you would expect that someone would be shocked and have a terrible reaction to such an event, yes or no?"

"Yes, that could certainly occur. But most people wouldn't react as extremely as Mrs. A. has."

"How can you know that?"

"I didn't say I know it as fact, just that I doubt most people would react as pathologically as Mrs. A. has."

"What do you mean by 'pathologically'?"

"I've already defined her pathology."

"Yes," interrupted Sanchez. "It's been asked and answered."

"You said most people would not react as pathologically as Mrs. A.," resumed Greenwood. "How do you *know* that?"

"I know it based on my training, education, and experience," I blurted out, realizing instantly I'd made a mistake by mentioning my training.

"Let's talk about your training, Doctor," Greenwood said, his eyes lasering on mine. "You're in the middle of your first year of residency, true?"

"Yes."

"So you've had about six months of training, correct?"

"Yes."

"So you still have a great deal to learn, don't you?"

"Yes."

"Yet you feel confident about the judgment you're making in this case?"

"I do. I've conferred with Dr. Jamison about Mrs. A."

"And in the six months of your training, how many patients have you seen who've lost a spouse in the traumatic way Mrs. A. has?"

"I haven't seen anyone with her situation."

"So how can you be sure that she's 'pathological,' to use your word?"

"When a patient can't work, when she's agitated and paces all day, when she mutters to herself and barely responds to questions, and when she's talking to a dead person, whom she says she will join soon, I know it's pathological."

"How do you know all this?"

"I've interviewed her every day since her admission. I've discussed her with Dr. Jamison. She's made some progress but needs more time to reintegrate. Right now she's very likely a danger to herself."

"And how do you know that?"

"Her mother heard her talking to her dead husband and is afraid she'll hurt herself."

"Did you interview her mother?"

"Yes. In the emergency room."

"How do you know her mother's a reliable historian?"

"She certainly sounded reliable and was very worried about her daughter. She described Patricia's condition and agreed she should come into the hospital."

"You *assumed* her mother's description to be accurate?"

"Yes, I did. In fact, before Patricia was brought to the hospital, she moved in with her mother."

"So you relied on what her mother told you?"

"Partly, yes. And it was confirmed by my examination of the patient."

"Doctor, a little while ago you said you examined Patricia in the emergency room, correct?"

"Yes."

"And she didn't talk?"

"That's correct."

"If she barely talked, how did you examine her?"

"Her not talking, her being unresponsive—basically, she was in a world of her own—was part of the findings. It was one of the *signs*—on examination."

"So, if a patient elects not to answer your questions, Doctor, you feel you have the right to deprive that person of her civil rights?"

"That's a gross oversimplification of what went on."

"But isn't that what it boils down to? She didn't answer your questions the way you deemed appropriate, so you threw her into the hospital."

"Not at all."

"Do you think we're in the Soviet Union?"[5]

"Objection!" shouted Sanchez. "That's irrelevant and absurd."

"The objection is sustained," said the judge.

"Isn't it true, Doctor, that Patricia is now talking and responds to questions, as opposed to your findings in the emergency room?"

"Yes. She's improving."

"Yet you feel she should still stay in the hospital?"

"Yes, she needs more time to get over the acute phase of this."

"Let me ask you, Doctor," Greenwood went on, barely pausing for breath. "Isn't it true that depression is often a temporary condition that can lift after a certain period of time?"

"That can happen."

"And the psychiatric community acknowledges that depression is often temporary, especially in *reactive* depressions, where the patient becomes depressed in *reaction* to a life event such as the one Patricia endured, correct?"

"Sometimes that's true—if the patient doesn't kill herself first."

"How can you be certain Patricia will harm herself if she's discharged?"

"I can't predict what she'll do, but there's still a good chance she wants to join her husband. Based on what I know from her history, after observing her behavior and evaluating her mental state, I feel there's a good likelihood she'll hurt herself if she's discharged now."

"But you don't *know* that, do you?"

"I can't say for certain that she will or she won't, only that there's a good chance it could happen."

---

5. This hearing took place before the breakup of the USSR.

"Again, Doctor, do you know it for a fact?"

"Not as a fact, no."

"Can you predict with any accuracy whether she will or will not harm herself?"

"I left my crystal ball at home, Mr. Greenwood."

Sanchez smothered a laugh. The judge remained neutral. I caught a glimpse of Patricia. She seemed to be glaring at me.

Greenwood shot me a veneer of a smile. "So, it's a judgment call on your part, isn't it?"

"Yes, it is."

"Has your judgment ever been wrong?"

"I'm sure it has."

"But you're certain it's not wrong with Patricia?"

"I think it's unlikely to be wrong."

"But you don't know for certain, do you?"

"A judgment call is what it is," I said. "You make a call based on all available evidence. There are very few absolute certainties in this life."

"Thank you for your philosophical musings, Doctor."

Sanchez piped up, "I object to Mr. Greenwood's snide remark, Your Honor."

"Sustained," said the judge. "Anything further, Mr. Greenwood?"

"I have no further questions," Greenwood said, shaking his head.

Judge Hobbs cleared his throat and looked squarely at me. "Doctor," he said, "what's your best judgment about Mrs. A.'s course of treatment?"

It was heartening to hear the judge use the word *judgment*.

"Dr. Jamison and I agree it's likely she'll improve over the next few weeks. Then she'll be transferred to the community ward, where she'll make more progress, and then be discharged. Afterward, she'll probably do well with outpatient treatment."

"So you view her ultimate prognosis as good?"

"Yes. It's very likely a good one."

"What makes you say that?"

"She's never been mentally ill before. She has a good work history. She's been a highly functioning person and has family support. It's likely she'll get back to her premorbid level of functioning."

"Going back to Mr. Greenwood's point about depression sometimes being temporary; is it likely Mrs. A. will improve without further treatment—and she'll get out of the state she's in right now?"

"The problem is, Your Honor, even if her depression is time-limited, while she's in this temporary state of mind, she could kill herself. If that happens, she'll have made a horrible decision with *permanent* consequences while she was in a *temporary* frame of mind. It's our obligation to protect her while she's in this temporary state."

The judge leaned back in his chair, nodded his head, and said, "Well put, Doctor." He paused and jotted a notation on the pad before him. He removed his glasses, set them on the table, and looked at Patricia A.

I'd been so focused on Greenwood, I hadn't noticed her for a while. Tears pooled in her eyes and then ran in runnels down her cheeks.

"Mrs. A.," the judge said. "What do you have to say?"

"I want to go home."

"Where would that be?" asked the judge.

"My mother's place."

"And what would you do there?"

She shook her head. "I don't know."

Greenwood leaned close to her and whispered something in her ear.

"Mrs. A.?" the judge asked. "Do you think you're ready to go back to work?"

She shrugged her shoulders.

"I know you've been through a difficult time," said the judge. "Do you feel ready to leave the hospital?"

"I just want to get out of here. I'm not crazy like the rest of these people. I just want to go home."

Tears dripped from her chin.

"Do you hear your husband's voice?" asked the judge.

She hesitated for a moment and then said, "No . . ."

"Are you being truthful, Mrs. A.?"

She nodded and sobbed. She dipped her head as her hands went to her face.

Judge Hobbs looked around the table. "Considering the testimony I've heard, and seeing Mrs. A. today, I think it's best if she stays in the hospital for the time being."

He turned to Greenwood. "If in two weeks you feel she doesn't require the hospital's protection, you can request another hearing, Mr. Greenwood. Until then we're obligated to protect Mrs. A. This hearing is concluded."

Chairs scraped on the linoleum floor as we rose. Sanchez shook my hand. "Congratulations," he whispered as we neared the dayroom doorway. "You handled Greenwood like a pro."

Three weeks later I visited Patricia on the open community ward, where she was being treated by another attending psychiatrist and resident.

At the nursing station, I read her chart. She was taking a powerful antidepressant, was undergoing counseling three times a week, and had improved substantially.

The community ward's dayroom was a large, cheerful expanse with chairs, two couches, and a small pool table. Potted geraniums and cacti lined the windowsills. A few patients were there. One was reading a book; another was knitting. Patricia was sitting on a sofa, thumbing through a magazine.

In contrast to her appearance when she was first admitted, she looked comfortable and relaxed. She'd gained back much of the weight she'd lost. She was dressed in jeans and a blouse and wore loafers. She smiled and stood to greet me.

"How are you feeling?" I asked.

"Much better. I feel . . . like there's hope for the future."

I felt a moment of deep satisfaction. It seemed Patricia might come to terms with her loss, negotiate the trauma she'd endured, and—despite everything—would go on with her life.

"I want to thank you," she said, smiling weakly.

"For what?" I replied, knowing I'd been a party to depriving her of her freedom.

"Just so you know," she whispered, "I listened to everything you said at the hearing."

"You needed a chance to begin healing."

"I understand," she said as tears shimmered in her eyes and a warm smile spread across her face. "Thank you for not letting me make a permanent decision in a temporary frame of mind."

Afterword

Some weeks later Patricia was discharged from the hospital. She continued outpatient sessions with the senior resident who had been treating her on the community ward. He told me she was doing quite well. Soon after discharge she went back to work and continued living with her mother until she found another apartment. The one in which she'd lived with Leonard held too many painful memories, and she was determined to move on with her life as best she could.

When the academic year ended in June, the resident left the hospital to establish a private practice, where he continued treating Patricia once weekly. He and I ran into each other occasionally at Grand Rounds and other professional gatherings. While confidentiality issues prevented him from going into detail, he said Patricia was doing very well—all things considered—and was making an excellent adjustment to her life as it had evolved.

Many patients have made an impact on me. Patricia is one of them. I sometimes wonder how she's doing all these years later. I still remember her words to me that day: "Thank you for not letting me make a permanent decision in a temporary frame of mind."

Patricia made a relatively quick recovery, which is unusual to see in the practice of psychiatry. We psychiatrists must often be satisfied with delaying the gratification a surgeon or an internist experiences when a patient improves dramatically.

In many medical specialties, conditions can be quickly eradicated or improved by a physician's timely intervention. Surgery, or medication, a one-time procedure, or physical manipulation may bring about rapid improvement or cure a physical problem.

But in psychiatry, progress is often delayed, sometimes for months or years. With psychotic patients, improvement may be rapid, but is often partial and only temporary. All too frequently, once they feel better, patients discontinue their medication and relapse into psychosis.

Other patients—those with bipolar disorder—often seem to hate being stabilized, preferring their manic highs, during which they feel ecstatic and are filled with boundless energy. They disregard the dangerous risk-taking behavior, impulsive decision-making, and financial or sexual promiscuity that accompanies these highs, preferring the manic state to the less intense reality of normalcy. So they discard their medication, and relapse invariably follows.

Treating people beset by neurotic problems can be difficult, frustrating, and time-consuming. Modifying a lifetime of maladaptive psychology is arduous work. Improvement, if it occurs, may be limited and can take years to achieve.

For psychiatrists, the gratification of seeing patients make meaningful progress is often delayed or never happens.

But it was different with Patricia and I will always remember her. She had decompensated completely and was probably going to commit suicide. It was gratifying to have played some part in her successfully negotiating a life-threatening mental illness.

And when I reflect back on that state-mandated hearing, I realize it was a seminal experience that sparked my interest in forensic psychiatry, the specialty I've practiced for many years.

A Man of Means

"Doctor, the police are here with a patient," the psychiatric ER reception clerk announced over the intercom.

Her voice conveyed a "you won't believe this" tone, that certain inflection everyone who worked in the ER knew signaled we were about to see a patient who presented in a very bizarre way. It was a common occurrence and most often meant someone suffering from a severe form of schizophrenia had arrived. Or it could be a patient with bipolar disorder whose disorganized speech flew in many different directions and constituted a form of word salad. The receptionist's tone led me to believe a "fascinoma" was here: a patient with psychopathology beyond anyone's comprehension—even for this place.

It was the 1980s, an era when the streets of New York City were filled with the dispirited, ragged, bedraggled, and homeless—part of the rotting underbelly of a city in decline, as it had been at the time. The police would often do what we called "dump-a-drunk." They'd drop some besotted soul off at the psychiatric emergency room rather than haul him to the precinct where he'd languish in the drunk tank. The police abhorred paperwork at least as much as we did and didn't want to deal with the hassle of a foul-smelling inebriate. But if the receptionist's tone of voice was in any way predictive, the new arrival wouldn't be a disorderly drunk.

Maybe it was someone whose family called the police, as often happened, when they knew a loved one was acting strangely and posed a danger to himself or others.

The police once brought in a man who'd been walking naked down the middle of 5th Avenue, or as happened in 1986, a homeless man who went berserk on the Staten Island Ferry, killing two people and wounding nine others with a sword, all the while proclaiming at the top of his lungs, "God's will be done" (the ultimate in command hallucinations). That poor deranged soul was brought to the hospital for evaluation while I was working in the emergency room.

I made my way to the waiting area. Sure enough, two cops sat in the gray plastic chairs, flanking a man.

I recognized Officer Frank Stark out of the 19th Precinct. We had a friendly but wary relationship. Though he usually ferried in people warranting hospitalization, he sometimes dragged in belligerent drunks who simply needed to sleep off an evening's overindulgence.

"You're on my turf now, Officer," I'd say, reminding him we weren't a drop zone for every booze-addled barfly who'd poured himself from a tavern only to be scraped off the streets.

"Hey, Doc," Stark said, extending his beefy hand. We shook hands and walked toward my office, leaving his partner babysitting the prospective patient. "We have an EDP for you, a really strange one."

EDP was police jargon for an emotionally disturbed person. But cops used that phrase promiscuously, expanding the definition to include intoxicated troublemakers.

"If he's another drunk, you'll be taking him to the precinct," I said, stifling a smile. It was hard to get angry at Stark. He was a good guy with a big heart.

But the emergency room was absolute bedlam. I'd already admitted eight patients, and on this warm Saturday night, the last thing we needed was a boisterous drunk cursing and splattering vomit.

"He's not drunk, Doc. He's an EDP, and believe me, this one's different."

"Different, how?" I asked, trying to rein in my skepticism.

"We got a call from Dispatch to proceed to the Regency Hotel. This guy was loitering in front of the hotel at the northwest corner of Park and Sixty-First. He was there for a good three hours."

"So . . . ?"

"When the doorman asked what he was doing, the guy said he was thinking of checking in to the *Regency*. Can you believe it? They thought he was off the wall. So the manager called the police."

"And then what?"

"When we arrived at the scene, he identified himself as *Mr. Smith*, but had no ID. Said he was thinking of taking a suite at the hotel. Get that—not a room, a *suite*, costing a few grand a night," Stark said, stifling a chortle. "He has this huge briefcase but won't let us look inside. He says he can pay the hotel's freight. We figured he should be seen here."

"Why'd you arrest him?"

"Loitering in a public place," Stark said, raising his hands. "He insists he's not a vagrant. Claims he has tons of money in the briefcase, but we can't open it. You know, Doc . . . the whole constitutional thing. We can't violate his civil rights." He shrugged his shoulders. "By the way, Doc, you get a look at him?"

"Not yet."

"There's no alcohol on his breath. What is it you guys say . . . no AOB? And his diction's clear . . . very clear. But you gotta get a load of this guy."

"Did you register him?"

"Yeah, as a John Doe. Get that . . . John Doe, aka Mr. Smith, wants a suite at the Regency."

"He's the third John Doe tonight."

"A busy night in the loony bin, huh?"

"As busy as the precinct."

Mr. Smith appeared at the office doorway.

My jaw may have dropped.

I'd never seen anyone looking quite as strange, yet paradoxically, there was also an air of normality about him.

He was of indeterminate age, perhaps in his fifties. He was a tall, cachectic-looking man whose face was so thin, he appeared cadaverous. His cheeks were hollow, which made his large eyes appear to be bulging from their sockets. Thick stubble with flecks of white covered his face and neck.

His curly hair was of medium length and graying at the temples. The room's fluorescent light cast a greenish hue over him.

He seemed like a ghostly apparition.

As striking as his skeletal look was, Mr. Smith's attire was remarkable. I'd never seen such clothing on a man who looked like he slept on sidewalk subway gratings.

He wore a soiled pin-striped, dark blue suit. The cut of cloth was undeniably high-end—maybe Brooks Brothers—but it had definitely seen better days. The edges of the sleeves were frayed. The lapels were curled and in need of ironing, as was the entire suit. The jacket and pants not only were wrinkled but sported a distinct sheen on the elbows and knees. His dress shirt had once been white but was now a soiled-looking off-gray. The collar was tattered, even threadbare. His suit hung from him like a circus tent, and his shirt collar was at least three sizes too large for his scrawny neck.

His ensemble was finished off with a dark blue silk tie, fashioned with a Windsor knot. It sported two dark stains a few inches below the fancy knot.

After closing the door, I sniffed subtly.

Officer Stark was right on the money: the man didn't smell of alcohol. Nor was there any odor of urea or acetone, surefire indications of metabolic pathology—impaired kidneys, liver, or pancreas.

"Have a seat, sir," I said, gesturing toward the chair facing my desk.

"Thank you," he answered in a resonant baritone voice.

"What's your name?" I asked, settling in behind my desk.

"You can call me Mr. Smith."

"What can I do for you, Mr. Smith?"

He looked at me with those globular, wet eyes and blinked a few times. "Why, thank you for taking the time to see me," he said in that mellifluous voice, so honeyed he sounded like a seasoned radio announcer.

I inhaled deeply, this time drawing the room's air into my lungs. Typically, when a vagrant sat in my tiny office, the room instantly filled with the stench of an unwashed body. But this time was different. There wasn't a trace of body odor.

And then, there was the bulging briefcase.

It was huge—obviously filled to the brim and latched shut. Its burgundy, marbled leather bespoke its origins, probably some high-end Madison Avenue shop frequented by Fortune 500 executives.

Mr. Smith clutched the tony briefcase tightly in his right hand.

Tucked neatly beneath his left arm was a folded copy of that day's *Wall Street Journal*.

Was it possible this man kept up with the financial news?

Sitting there, he looked about the office, as though sizing it up. I couldn't tell if he was aggrieved to be in the psychiatric emergency room. After all, he'd been hauled in presumably against his will by two cops in a squad car.

Was Mr. Smith psychotic, an eccentric millionaire, or simply an itinerant soul needing a place to bed down for the night? Or was something else beyond my imaginings going on?

He sat quietly, appeared composed, and some moments later set his briefcase on the floor beside him.

His movements were fluid and graceful as he crossed one leg over the other, revealing charcoal-gray hose and black wing-tipped shoes.

It was all so incongruous: he appeared daintily fastidious and exuded an aura of cultured refinement; but his threadbare clothing and dire circumstances suggested something had gone terribly wrong.

What was his story?

A torrent of diagnostic possibilities shuttled through my mind.

Was this man some Wall Street honcho who'd seen better days? An out-of-work broker or bond trader whose financial world had collapsed? Had he been embroiled in a money-sapping divorce that drained him of spirit *and* cash—leaving him broken, bedraggled, and confused? Was he a member of some prestigious corporate board who'd been shunted aside in an internal reshuffling, resulting in his becoming delusional? Or maybe he'd been with some white-shoe law firm, perhaps even as a partner, and had been forced to resign.

Or, was he a street-dwelling charlatan who'd snatched an expensive briefcase and was wearing a suit retrieved from some back-alley Dumpster?

Or, as unlikely as it seemed, did he have sufficient cash to secure a suite at the Regency Hotel?

The door of another office opened and slammed against the tile wall. A man's screaming could be heard. "How dare you!" cried the voice. "You can't do this to me. I'm Jesus Christ!"

A commotion followed. Nurses and attendants could be heard running, and the sounds of a struggle followed. "You can't treat me this way. I'm the Savior!"

Mr. Smith sat calmly. His huge eyes stared directly at me. There was no muscle twitching or tightening of facial muscles, or any other indication he was cognizant of the commotion outside. If he was, it didn't faze him at all.

"I'm here to save you all!" "Jesus" roared, and from the decreasing decibel level, it was clear he'd been tied down in a high-backed wheelchair and was being trundled toward an elevator to be taken upstairs.

Mr. Smith simply sat in place, unruffled.

"What brings you here?" I said.

"May I smoke?" He produced a gold-plated cigarette case. I'd only seen them in old movies.

Back then smoking was allowed in hospitals. I shoved the metal ashtray on the desktop closer to him.

His slender fingers gingerly extracted a cigarette from the case. I was struck by his clean, neatly trimmed nails—rarely seen when a vagrant sat in the office.

With a gold-plated lighter, he lit up.

He inhaled and exhaled contrails of smoke through his nostrils. His entire manner bespoke gentility.

"So . . . what brings you here?" I repeated. I wasn't impatient; I was achingly curious.

"Well, sir, I'm looking for a place to stay. It's been a trying time for me." He gazed up at the ceiling and took another drag on his cigarette. His hand movements were refined, almost delicate, as he tapped his cigarette on the ashtray's lip.

"What kind of place are you looking for?" I asked, truly perplexed.

"What kind of place am I looking for?" he responded dreamily. "I'm not sure, but the accommodations must be suitable, preferably with a well-stocked minibar and excellent room service. I'm finicky about cleanliness."

"I see," I said, not really knowing where to take this line of questioning. The man was a complete paradox. None of this made any sense.

"And I need peace and quiet," he added. "I've been under a good deal of stress and want to relax, not be disturbed."

"I understand you were at the Regency Hotel. What were you doing there?"

"Assessing the clientele."

"What for?"

"To determine if I'd feel comfortable sharing accommodations with them."

"Would you?"

"Probably, although you know how standards have dropped these days. There are so few people with social graces."

He smiled. Was he being serious or toying with me?

His right eye nearly closed, as if he were winking. But it could have been a facial tic. The eyelid remained at half-mast for a moment and then opened. He examined the lit end of his cigarette and then peered at me, as though inviting another question.

"Tell me, Mr. Smith, how did things used to be for you?" I tried imagining the trajectory of this man's life.

"I'm not sure I can go into that right now," he said, looking away.

I must have tapped into something of great meaning to him.

"Why not?"

"An injudicious word could result in repercussions. I don't want to say something that could be considered defamatory. You know, about insider trading or other felonies forbidden by the SEC."

"Are you an attorney or involved with some financial institution?"

"No, though I've thought of going into arbitrage and investment banking. But it's a bit underhanded, if you know what I mean. The law is certainly one of my interests. You might even say it's an avocation. But I hold no great affection for lawyers—actually, none at all. They're a detestable breed, by and large."

Though formal and stilted, his speech was clear and coherent. Each word followed logically from the one preceding it and led seamlessly to the next. There was no sign of a speech disorder or cognitive impairment. His evasiveness was in the service of protecting himself from imagined or real enemies, adversaries, or defamatory liability.

But was it persecutory? Was he paranoid? Or merely being judicious?

And that *voice*—incredibly mellow—a stage actor's voice, or that of a radio announcer on a classical music station like WQXR. And his vocabulary wasn't the street patois you'd typically hear in the psychiatric emergency room. His choice of words was more suited to the upper-crust Metropolitan Club.

Gazing about the office, he took in the overhead fluorescent light, the battered wooden desk, the off-white tile walls, and the sickly looking greenish linoleum floor. Flicking more ash from his cigarette, he said, "This looks like a clean establishment. How much do you charge for a night's stay?"

I was stunned. He'd gone from perusing the Regency Hotel to querying me about the nightly rate for a room at *Manhattan Hospital*? And this was asked by a freakishly fastidious guy who valued cleanliness, peace, and quiet.

Cleanliness?

His clothing would be turned down by the Salvation Army.

Peace and quiet? The psychiatric hospital wards were modern-day versions of Bedlam.

"I'm not sure you'd want to stay *here*, Mr. Smith."

"Why not?" His eyes questioned me with bulbous curiosity.

"Well, a man of your caliber . . ."

"Oh, I'm not a snob, if that's what you think."

"No, not at all. But I don't know if this place would meet your standards."

"That's yet to be determined."

"Mr. Smith, do you know where you are?"

"Of course."

"Where are we?"

"Oh, my good man, let's not get into absurdities. You and I are discussing whether or not I'd like to stay at your facility. There's no need to be insulting."

His Adam's apple bobbed up and down. He'd managed to make me feel like a complete jerk.

"Or perhaps it's a matter of money, because that's what so many things reduce to in this sad world." He made a *tsk* sound, inserted the cigarette delicately between his lips, and sucked inward. More streams of smoke trailed from his nostrils. "Yes, it's a sad world where greed rules. Maybe you think I lack the funds to cover a stay at your facility," he said as his forehead furrowed.

"Well, a stay here can be pretty expensive," I replied, thinking it was both absurd and sensible to be talking this way. The going rate back then for an inpatient stay at Manhattan Psychiatric was quite formidable. The daily rate charged to Medicare and Medicaid was stratospheric, and it didn't include doctors' bills or special studies like X-rays, CT scans, or things like ECT (electro-convulsive therapy), medications, and sundries.

"Let me assure you, Doctor, I can cover the fee."

My eyes involuntarily sought out the bulging briefcase.

"I'm a man of means," he stated, pausing as if to emphasize the point. "A man of *substantial* means, no matter what my circumstances suggest now. As a matter of fact, despite the recent downturn in the markets, I'm quite comfortable."

I hoped my poker face didn't reveal my skepticism. I always tried to appear nonjudgmental when dealing with emergency-room patients. You never knew how a momentary look of doubt or disbelief could set off an eruption of madness.

"I can see you have doubts," he said, stubbing his cigarette in the ashtray. "Let me assure you my portfolio is quite substantial. I have a well-diversified mixture of assets. It's very balanced among various instruments, and no matter what the markets do on any given day or week—or month for that matter—I'm quite well positioned."

"I see . . ."

"You should be aware that, among other precautionary tactics, I've been dollar-cost averaging in an array of diversified mutual funds. And my other investments—bonds of all sorts—are laddered over time so the maturity dates are always coming due. It allows for a comfortable cash flow and excellent liquidity."

He began talking about PE ratios, stock splits, short selling, hedging, and other fiscal tactics, some arcane, others more commonplace. Then he launched into a tsunami of verbiage about the Russell 5000, the Dow, and the S&P 500.

His knowledge of the financial world was astonishing. Clearly he was a man of intellectual heft and fiscal sophistication. As for his alleged finances, who could know?

I grew even more curious about the contents of that bulging briefcase. Was it stuffed with bearer bonds?

With a horde of cash?

Or some other asset of great value?

One thing was apparent: he'd obviously seen better times. Was there a reasonably plausible chance he'd managed to stash away a ton of money at some point in his life, despite his psychiatric condition, whatever it was?

And who could know what stresses he'd been under? I again wondered if he was on the wrong end of some devastating corporate feud leaving him compromised to the point of being a cash-rich vagrant. How could I, or anyone for that matter, know the life-altering crises leading to his sitting in this dingy little office at a hospital's psychiatric emergency room? Every patient had a story to tell. What was *this* man's personal arc—his own strange trajectory? By what serpentine route had his life funneled down to this sad yet dignified path he now traveled? What dire chain of events led to his awaiting my verdict about his admissibility to a psychiatric ward?

"Recently, I was forced to liquidate certain holdings," he continued. "But the bulk of my portfolio is intact. Some of what I cashed out is here with me."

"You mean in the briefcase?"

"Yes," he said, staring directly into my eyes.

"Is that cash you're carrying around?"

"Yes. It's enough to cover a stay at any establishment."

"How much money is in there?"

His eyes narrowed. "Why do you ask, sir?"

"Well, carrying lots of cash around the city isn't a good idea."

"Oh, it's a goodly sum," he said, glancing at the briefcase.

"It can be dangerous to walk the streets with so much cash."

"Perhaps. But I assume your establishment has a safe where I could store this if I decide to stay."

"Yes. We store belongings when we admit someone to this facility."

"You said *admit* someone. I'm impressed. It sounds like you're selective."

"Well, Mr. Smith, we do have certain criteria for admission," I said, wondering just where—if anyplace—Mr. Smith fit on the spectrum of mental illness. Was he psychotic? Delusional in the steadfast belief he had tons of money, when in fact he was a street-dwelling pauper? Was I being strung along by a man who presented himself as conversant in fiscal and corporate machinations but had nothing in the way of assets? Was he a former actor, a radio announcer, a corporate honcho or an attorney; or was he simply a charlatan enjoying his little charade?

"I like that you have criteria for choosing clientele," Mr. Smith said. A smile of satisfaction crossed his face. "So . . . you're selective."

"You could say that," I replied, knowing our selectivity involved lawfully mandated criteria—we admitted only psychotic people whose illnesses rendered them dangerous to themselves or others.

"Let me assure you I can pay *whatever* the going rate is," he stressed. "I could pay on a day-by-day basis, or settle up each month, in advance. In cash, if you prefer. I assume you have long-term guests?"

"Yes, a select few."

"Perhaps we could consider such an arrangement." Those eyes grew wider with every question.

"To tell you the truth, Mr. Smith, I'm not really sure."

"Do you doubt my fiscal integrity?"

He leaned back in his chair and squinted. I thought momentarily he might wink again, but nothing of the sort happened. Rather, his lips turned down. "Because if you have doubts, I can dispel them completely, right now."

He reached for the briefcase.

My pulse quickened. This could be the curtain-closer—the great reveal. I leaned forward to see the satchel.

He pulled it from the floor to his lap.

I was again struck by its pebbled, reddish brown leather texture, by its heft and obvious weight as it sat on his thin thighs. It was all so strange—the expensive but decrepit sartorial ensemble, accompanied by his fiscal verbiage and stilted speech. It was comical and sad, borderline believable, yet farcical, and above all, impossible to understand.

"You know," he said, "the federal government stopped issuing thousand-dollar bills in 1969."

"Really? Since 1969?" I asked, humoring him.

"Yes. Because of money laundering, President Nixon issued an executive order limiting the printing of denominations to a maximum of one-hundred-dollar bills. It's too bad, because it makes carrying large sums of cash quite onerous."

He snapped open the latches. I estimated the case weighed at least thirty pounds, probably more. He repositioned it on his lap.

"Are you sure you want to open that?" I asked.

He shifted the case to his arms as he rose from the chair. "I simply want to dispel any doubts you may have about my fiscal integrity."

He turned and set the briefcase on the chair, his back to me as he bent over it. "I'll show you some of the liquidated portion of my portfolio."

Mr. Smith peered into the now-open briefcase. He nodded and turned slowly toward me with the satchel—open at the top. He cradled the thing, almost lovingly.

I sat behind the desk, waiting expectantly, aware of the steady hum of fluorescent lights.

A smile crossed Mr. Smith's face as he began tilting the brief-case forward. Its open end hovered over the desktop.

He was going to dump its contents onto the desk.

I leaned back, waiting in anticipation. My pulse quickened, feeling like a drumbeat in my neck.

Just how much pure, hard, cold cash was Mr. Smith toting around New York City? Just how risky was this absurd odyssey, given the high crime rate—the holdups and muggings—the innumerable dangers of the city streets?

The briefcase hung over the desk.

He began turning it upside down.

My heart thrashed violently.

Then, as though it were a waterfall, cash began pouring forth—bundles and bundles of tightly wrapped money. And then more packs dumping, slapping heavily onto the wooden desktop.

It was an avalanche of paper. Each large bundle—maybe three inches thick—was neatly bound with a red rubber band.

There were wrapped stacks of hundred-dollar bills, with at least fifty or a hundred bills to a pack—a good five to ten thousand dollars in each tightly banded bundle. And there were dozens upon dozens of bundles, even a few hundred packets, more than my eyes could register at the moment—pouring forth from the briefcase's open end.

The landslide of money was stupendous.

As the shock of the deluge dissipated, I immediately noticed something: each one-hundred-dollar bill at the top of every banded bundle was emblazoned with a huge "100" within a circle.

At the upper-right corner of each bill was the silhouette of a locomotive, while a picture at the lower left corner depicted a house.

Every bill of this heaped hoard of cash, each finely printed, pale *yellow* one-hundred-dollar bill was but a small part of an enormous aggregate of a few million dollars—*all in Monopoly money*.

My eyes must have bulged even more than Mr. Smith's. Nearly paralytic, I gazed at this incredible stash of cash; then, as disbelief flooded me, I looked up at the man standing before me.

As he stared at the mountain of ersatz wealth, Mr. Smith's face radiated a smile of profound satisfaction. I could actually *feel* his sense of accomplishment at having amassed this board-game fortune.

"You see, sir, I'm well financed. I have much more in a locker at Penn Station."

My head was nearly spinning.

"Mr. Smith, will you wait here for a moment?" I said as I got up from my chair. "Actually, why don't you put your money back in the briefcase."

"I assume you can arrange for my accommodations . . ."

"I'll do my best," I said, realizing Stark was right: this was no ordinary case. This was no foul-mouthed drunkard shouting vitriolic curses at people on the city streets. This was no stench-ridden bench-clearer on the Lexington Avenue subway, or a Bible-shouting proselytizer ranting on Park Avenue. Mr. Smith or Doe, or whatever his real name might be, was no raving lunatic.

But he was certainly delusional and disturbed.

"Could you arrange for a room with a view?" he asked.

"I'll try, Mr. Smith."

He began scooping up the bundles and dumped them into the briefcase.

I excused myself and left the office.

"Well, Doc, whaddaya think?" Sergeant Stark asked in the reception area. "What's the story with him?"

"I'm not sure, but we'll do our best to find out. I'll make arrangements for him to check into our accommodations momentarily."

"Everyone's got a story to tell, right, Doc?"

"Yup. Everyone has a story."

"Hey, ever find out what's in the briefcase?"

"Yeah. He has some money," I said, knowing if I revealed the contents of the briefcase, Stark would break out laughing. There was something about Mr. Smith's inherent dignity that precluded me from making his madness the butt of humor.

"Really. How much?"

"Not much. But we'll take care of him for a while."

"Saves me a ton of paperwork, Doc."

"And ours is about to begin."

"Will you sign this paper?" he asked, producing a release form. "It just says you accept custody."

"Sure," I said, slipping a pen from my pocket and nodding to a huge white-coated male attendant. "He won't require any restraints," I said as the attendant neared the office door. "And I'll do the physical exam when he's settled in upstairs. Just give me a call."

Knowing exactly what I meant, the attendant summoned another gargantuan guy. They proceeded into the office.

"Good evening, Mr. Smith," I heard the first attendant say.

"Good evening, gentlemen," came the reply. "I assume you'll

show me to my room."

"Sure, Mr. Smith. We'll take you upstairs."

And so Mr. Smith checked into a room at the Manhattan "Hotel." At least for a few days and nights, if not longer.

I wondered if, with a little time and conversation, we would learn more about his story.

After all, everyone has a story to tell.

Afterword

Since he was no longer my patient but would be the responsibility of the psychiatrists on the locked men's ward, I knew the physical examination would be my last opportunity to learn more, firsthand, about Mr. Smith.

When I entered his room, he greeted me with the same cordiality he'd exhibited in the ER.

He thanked me for my hospitality. It didn't seem to register with him that this *hospitality* was being delivered in a psychiatric hospital, not some luxury hotel.

As the physical exam proceeded, he expressed delight at being given such luxurious treatment. It was as if he were in a spa, not a psych ward.

Try as I might, I was unable to divert his conversation away from the excellent accommodations and services he was receiving.

After making the appropriate entry into his chart, I returned to the ER, frustrated but with piqued curiosity.

While I knew it would be difficult to locate records, the Monopoly money was a good lead.

Those were the days before computers and e-mail. Over the next week, I telephoned a few psychiatric emergency rooms and managed to obtain some sketchy information.

Records indicated a man fitting Mr. Smith's description, and carrying a briefcase stuffed with ersatz money, had visited various hospitals. Each time he used a different name.

Most physicians diagnosed Mr. Smith as a paranoid man with delusions of grandeur. Only one took seriously his claims about having once worked on Wall Street.

I tracked down that doctor, a psychiatric resident at Roosevelt Hospital, who said he, too, had been intrigued by "Mr. Wilber Grant," when he examined him one year earlier. Mr. Grant told him he'd worked as an account executive at Bear Stearns.

But after some telephone calls to the investment house's personnel and human resources departments, the resident said his inquiry came up empty: no one by that name, or even remotely resembling the patient, had ever worked in any of their offices.

Maybe he'd been a highly functioning executive.

Maybe the suit had been tailor-made, fitting properly and pristinely pressed, at a far better time in his life.

Maybe the briefcase was a gift from a loving wife after he'd become a partner at a law firm.

Maybe he and his wife (if he'd had one) were divorced, which had thrown him into the abyss of homelessness and madness.

Maybe the expensive briefcase, cigarette case, and lighter were trappings of a life once lived in luxury.

Maybe the cultured tones and gracious manner were products of an education from the finest private schools and an Ivy League campus.

Or maybe none of my imaginings ever happened.

There was simply no way to find out.

All these years later, I'm still intrigued by these questions.

It's really quite ironic. I fell in love with psychiatry because each patient—though sharing human commonalities—had a uniquely personal story.

While everyone has a story to tell, not everyone will tell his story.

Some stories end happily, others in tragedy.

And some end on a note of uncertainty.

A Dirty Little Secret

Some symptoms can alter patients' daily experiences so profoundly that their lives become unlivable. Yet despite the severity of these conditions, they may not warrant psychiatric hospitalization.

Anyone who's been plagued by bouts of anxiety, an occasional panic attack, a smoldering, joy-sapping depression, or an irrational phobia can attest to a simple fact: unless symptoms become unbearable or pervasive, most people don't go for help. They struggle through each day, living as Thoreau put it, "lives of quiet desperation."

But the sudden onset of a powerful symptom can upend one's life; and only when the symptom intensifies to the breaking point may the affected person seek help.

Barbara C. was forty-three years old, and after a year of escalating symptoms, finally came to the clinic for a psychiatric consultation.

An attractive woman, she wore a starched white blouse, a beige skirt, and high-heeled shoes. Her lipstick was a rich crimson color and her eyeshadow and liner had been meticulously applied. But most striking was the jet-black hair cascading to her shoulders. Her look was vaguely reminiscent of movie starlets from the 1950s.

"I think I'm going crazy," she began, sitting down and adjusting her skirt over her knees.

"What makes you say that?" I asked, knowing patients sometimes found symptoms so strange and frightening, they could begin doubting their sanity.

"I think I'm having a nervous breakdown. I may have to come into the hospital." She seemed to be shivering. "I just can't control myself."

"What can't you control?"

She sighed and closed her eyes. "About a year ago, I discovered something . . ." She stopped midsentence. She was clearly reluctant to discuss whatever she'd unearthed. Was her husband having an affair? Was she under threat of something terrible happening in her life?

"What did you discover?"

She shook her head, looked away, and said nothing.

Frequently, patients needed gentle prodding to talk about their symptoms or reveal their innermost thoughts and fantasies. To talk openly about their troubles is mortifying for some people.

Barbara's facial muscles tightened; the corners of her mouth turned down.

After a long pause, she began. "God, this sounds so vain. I'm embarrassed to talk about it . . ." She closed her eyes, sighed, and then a moment later continued. "One morning I looked in the mirror and saw a patch of white hair right on the top of my head, near the front. I'd never noticed it before. It seemed to have happened overnight."

She fell silent and looked away into a nonexistent distance.

It was doubtful a patch of white hair made a sudden appearance. More likely, she'd only noticed it that particular morning, which made me wonder what happened to make her so exquisitely conscious of her appearance. True, she was meticulously groomed, with an obvious sense of style, but my antennae told me far more was afoot than the appearance of some white hair. No, there was something deeper troubling her.

As she sat before me, it was obvious she'd dyed the offending patch; her hair was uniformly raven black.

"I just can't control it," she began again.

"I'm not sure I understand," I said. "What can't you control?"

"I don't know why it worried me so much, but when I saw that white hair, I nearly went out of my mind. I ran out and bought some hair dye. I applied it according to the instructions. But then I noticed I'd gotten some dye on my hands. The skin was discolored, so I washed my hands, but it wouldn't come off. I washed them again, but the dye was still there."

She looked down at her hands and squinted.

"And when I looked very carefully, I realized some dye was on the towel I'd used to dry my hands. So I threw the towel in the washing machine. When I took it out, the spot was a little lighter, but it was still there."

I imagined the sequence of events that followed. This could very well be the beginning of an obsessive thought, a recurrent idea that would intrude into consciousness and on which she would focus insistently, no matter how valiantly she would try to banish it.

"What happened then?"

"It got worse . . ."

"How?"

"Not only were my hands and the towel stained, but I realized the dye got into the washing machine. I only thought of it after I'd done a few loads of wash, and I was convinced I got dye onto everything I'd washed in the machine."

"So, you couldn't stop thinking about dye getting on everything?"

"Yes. I was convinced it got onto all the clothes, that it was everywhere."

I couldn't help but think of Lady Macbeth's words. *"Out, damned spot! Out, I say!"*

"The stain was spreading." Her lower lip began quivering. "I was worried that everything I touched was stained, like it was contaminated. I know this sounds ridiculous," she said, putting her palm to her cheek, "and I'm not a stupid person, but it just kept getting worse."

"So you knew this idea didn't make sense," I said, trying to assess her awareness of how irrational her symptom had become.

"Yes, I knew it then, and I know it now. But I couldn't control it. If I didn't do another load of wash, I'd start pacing and worrying about the dye. I'd imagine it on all the clothing, in the drawers, everywhere. I couldn't stop worrying about it. And my heart would race a mile a minute. The only thing that calmed me down was doing the laundry again."

Barbara was describing a compulsion—an uncontrollable urge to repeat unproductive, time-consuming behavior again and again—in the service of trying to undo an obsessive thought.

"But it got worse," she continued, shifting in the chair. "I began thinking everything was contaminated . . . that it had spread through the house. I started scrubbing the kitchen floor—every day. And then vacuuming the carpets, the drapery, and venetian blinds, the sofa, chairs, everything."

"Did that help?"

"No," she said, as a sob nearly burst from her throat. She clutched her elbows and bent forward. Her face turned pasty white. "After I was through cleaning, I'd feel better for a while, but there was always more. So, I'd start all over again . . . the laundry, the house . . . even me."

"You mean the dye on your hands?"

"Not just my hands, my whole body. I began showering two or three times a day. My skin got dry and flaky. So I used lotion and then worried the cream was dirty, that maybe some dye got into it. I couldn't get clean, no matter what I did."

She paused and squinted. A latticework of fine lines appeared around her eyes.

"Then I had this idea—I know it sounds crazy—this idea . . . that if I touched money, I'd get more filth on me, because you never know where money's been."

It was like the proverbial ripples spreading outward from a stone tossed into a placid lake; her symptoms were expanding through every facet of her life.

"So I sent my husband out shopping. He went along with it for a while, but he works long hours. And now he's losing patience with me; he won't tolerate it. He comes home from work tired and wants to relax, and there I am, worried and nervous. I mean . . . he's a good man—we've been married for twenty-one years—and I love him. I don't want my marriage to end. He convinced me to come for help."

"It's good you did," I said.

"This is some kind of phobia, isn't it? It's a dirt phobia, right? That's what my friend said."

"Yes, and the need to clean everything is called a compulsion. It's something you feel you *have* to do. If you don't do it, you feel nervous. And by cleaning, you get some temporary relief."

She nodded, almost frantically, and then clasped her hands around her knees. She was nearly rocking back and forth.

"Can you help me?" she asked with widened eyes.

"Yes, I think we can help you. But first I'd like—"

"Because I can't go on this way. It's unbearable. And my husband . . . I don't know how much more he can take."

People like Barbara often live with their symptoms until they become unbearable, or begin undermining key relationships, like Barbara's with her husband.

"We'll do our best to help. But I'd like to understand a little more. You said this began about a year ago?"

"Yes."

"What was going on then?"

"Nothing I can think of." She looked away. Her eyes were unfocused.

"Are you sure? Take a moment to think about it."

Her brow formed a V-shaped crease. "There was nothing. I just woke up one morning and saw that white patch."

"Think back to that morning. What happened?"

"I got out of bed. My husband left early for a business meeting in Boston. I slept a bit later than usual because we'd been out the night before, but there was nothing different about that morning."

"You said you'd been out late the night before. What did you do?"

"Oh, that? It was no big deal," she said with a dismissive wave of her hand.

"What was no big deal?"

"Oh, it was ridiculous. I'm embarrassed to even mention it."

"Embarrassed about what?"

"It was nothing . . ."

It must have been something, I thought, because she was doing her utmost to avoid talking about it.

"Tell me about it."

We might be getting close to pay dirt.

She peered at the floor. I could almost detect her cerebral gears in motion.

"Oh, we went to my twenty-fifth high school reunion. Don't ever go to those things," she added, looking away. Then she let out a soft laugh. "All you see are people who've gotten old. You picture them from when they were eighteen, and when you get there, what do you see? A bunch of middle-aged people you hardly recognize. It's like your whole life's been fast-forwarded. The men have huge bellies. And most of them have no hair, which they try to disguise with those horrible comb-overs.

"And the women . . . My God, what happens to people as they go through life is so pathetic." She shook her head, closed her eyes, and then shrugged. "But who looks like they did twenty-five years ago?"

"It sounds like seeing your old classmates bothered you."

"No. Actually, it made me feel better about myself. I don't look like I've been through the meat grinder the way so many of them did. I've taken care of myself. Before this dirt thing began, I went to the gym nearly every day. Used the treadmill, swam, and even lifted light weights." She again crossed her arms in front of herself. "No, seeing them didn't make me feel older. I felt good about myself. In fact . . ." Her voice trailed off and she fell silent.

"What just happened?"

"What do you mean?"

"You were about to say something. You said, 'In fact,' and then stopped."

Something had intruded into her thoughts, made her stop dead in her tracks.

She looked contemplative and then began blinking frequently. Her eyes looked wet.

"Is there something on your mind right now?"

"Not really."

I'd long ago learned when a patient says *not really*, it means something is *really* being avoided, something the patient *really* doesn't want to discuss.

After a long pause, I said, "You were saying you felt good about yourself at the reunion. And you were about to say something, but it slipped away."

She sighed. "There was one thing . . ."

I waited. We sat in silence for a few moments. I held back from pushing too hard. But what was that *one thing*?

"Well, there was . . ." Her voice grew softer. "I saw Jack there." More silence.

I waited, sensing we were getting close to something meaningful.

She sighed. "He was my boyfriend during my junior and senior years of high school."

The room was very quiet.

"How was that for you?" I asked.

She straightened up in the chair. "Oh God, time just telescoped. I might as well have been back in high school, you know . . . at the prom. But I wasn't. It was twenty-five years later at the Grand Hyatt in Manhattan. And I felt—I don't know . . . I was very self-conscious. He was the only man there who wasn't overweight, bald, and old-looking. He was as handsome as ever, just more mature-looking with a touch of white hair at his temples."

She sighed again.

"What did you feel self-conscious about?"

She shrugged. "Oh, you know . . . I was very aware of him looking at me. I mean, he was there with his wife—who wasn't a winner. And I was there with Walter, my husband. Jack and I didn't really talk much, but I knew the old fire was still there."

She pursed her lips and closed her eyes for a moment.

"And I felt—I don't know—I just thought a lot about him on the way home and when I was lying in bed that night. I couldn't stop thinking about the old times, back in the day, you know? It brought back lots of memories from twenty-five years ago, when things were different."

She looked away and then turned to me and said, "It could be a century later, and you know what? The flame never dies. Not completely."

"Do you mean Jack's flame or your own?"

"I—I guess both of us. I mean, I felt this weird static while we were talking. He felt the same way. I could tell. We stood off to the side while Walter and Jack's wife were talking. And my heart was racing. I felt goose bumps all over me. It was almost like an alarm went off the moment I saw him. It was something deep inside me.

For a couple of years back in high school, I thought he was the love of my life. But I was a kid. What do kids know?"

"So what happened to the two of you after senior year?"

"Oh, we each went off to college, and you know . . . we went our separate ways. Pretty typical, isn't it?"

I remained silent.

Her eyes narrowed. "You think this has something to do with Jack, don't you?"

"What makes you say that?"

"You asked about him. That's how we got onto this whole thing."

"I only asked what happened the evening before you noticed the patch of white hair that morning."

She nodded. It was unclear if she understood the implication of what had just occurred.

"So, do you think you can help me?"

It was solid gold. She'd evaded an attempt to probe more about the reunion—and the feelings evoked by seeing Jack for the first time in twenty-five years. But she'd said enough.

It was a clinical certainty: when a patient deflected a topic or question, it was in the service of avoiding a deeper, more meaningful truth. One she didn't want to discuss.

Did some fantasy surface about Jack—from time lost but now recalled? Had seeing Jack reignited that old flame, making her feel guilty? Had it made her suddenly feel old—so she noticed a white patch of hair the next morning and decided to push back the clock?

Had seeing Jack caused some forbidden wish to surface, one so threatening she had to wash it away? After all, her heart had been racing and she'd felt goose bumps when she once again saw the love of her life. Had the reunion evoked her awareness of buried regrets? Was her marriage to Walter as satisfying as she claimed? Maybe seeing Jack was a forbidden chance to relive the past in the here and now, at least in a forbidden fantasy.

Had this yearning threatened to contaminate her life, her marriage? Did she have to undo that dirty little secret by compulsive, ritualistic cleansing of her body and home?

I found myself thinking of patients described by Freud and the Viennese psychoanalysts at the turn of the twentieth century.

But it wasn't 1909, and we weren't in Vienna.

And Barbara C. wasn't ready for a deeply probing exploration of forbidden wishes or fantasies. Instead, she would do everything possible to push them away, to negate them, to cleanse herself and the home in which she lived with her husband, benighted Walter.

Besides, it could take a long time to help her unearth such taboo thoughts and feelings. Most patients visiting a psychiatrist come for relief, and that was Barbara's motivation—to alleviate the symptomatic horror her life had become.

So, do you think you can help me? was her question.

"Yes, you can be helped," I said.

She closed her eyes. "Oh, thank you. What will help?"

"There are medications for treating your symptoms. We can start with one of them."

"Which medication?"

"There's Paxil or Zoloft—"

"Aren't they for depression?"

"Yes, and they're also used to treat your symptoms—the hand washing, the nervousness, the phobia . . ."

"Which one will you use?"

"You know this is only a consultation. I won't be treating you, but you'll be assigned to someone here at the clinic."

"Will you be in touch with whoever it is?"

"Yes, definitely. We'll talk about starting you on some medication, probably Paxil, at a very low dose."

"Is it addictive?"

"No, not at all."

"Will I have to stay on it for the rest of my life?"

"Probably not. The idea is to smother the symptoms—the worries about dye and dirt and all the washing and cleaning. After a few months, your therapist will begin tapering the medication."

"The symptoms . . . will they come back?"

"We can't know right now. But you and your therapist will meet and see if you can understand why this began. Meanwhile, we can suffocate the symptoms, and you can get back to your normal life, the way things were before you woke up that morning."

"So you still think the reunion started this, don't you?" Her eyes narrowed.

There was nothing to be gained by denying or confirming her suspicion—one she attributed solely to me.

Instead, I said, "I'll be talking with your therapist later today, and while you're in treatment, you'll look into the reunion and what it meant to you. But first we'll try to get things back on an even keel."

Afterword

Barbara was seen regularly by her clinic therapist. After six weeks at a moderately low dose of medication, her obsessional ideas and the compulsive need to cleanse everything were suffocated. She was able to resume a reasonably normal life.

Over the next year, I kept in touch with her therapist, who reported Barbara's obsessional ideas returned whenever the dose was lowered. When raised to its former level, Barbara continued on symptom-free.

During her second year in treatment at the psychopharmacology clinic, still symptom-free and by then, on a very low dose of medication—basically a placebo level—Barbara abruptly terminated therapy.

When her therapist asked her about this, she was evasive. She said she would continue receiving prescriptions for the medication from her family doctor.

Shortly thereafter the therapist called her home to clarify an issue on an insurance form. Walter answered and told the psychiatrist that Barbara had left him.

Was my colleague shocked by this revelation?

Not really.

He described the situation very well, saying, "Barbara was very good at keeping secrets, even from herself."

Did she try resuming her relationship with Jack?

Probably. After all, she'd constructed an enduring fantasy in her mind—he was the love of her life—and maybe she could return to the halcyon days of her youth.

Would her obsessive-compulsive disorder return?

That was unknowable, especially since Barbara was unwilling to explore the reasons for her dirty little secret.

Virtually everyone has occasional obsessive thoughts and engages in trivial compulsive behaviors. Haven't we all, as children, walked along a sidewalk and avoided stepping on a crack? How many of us have counted telephone poles or other routine objects during the course of a day? Hasn't each of us occasionally wondered if a door is locked or a gas jet turned off? At times we each have felt a compelling need to check or recheck something—the alarm clock setting or some other minor object or task.

That's not obsessive-compulsive disorder.

Some years ago, obsessive-compulsive disorder (OCD) was thought to be rare. But in fact it's really quite a bit more common than formerly believed. "I know I'm not crazy, but what I'm doing is crazy, and I can't stop it!" is a typical complaint of someone truly suffering from OCD. That's how Barbara presented.

For OCD to be diagnosed, obsessions and/or compulsions must be a real source of distress; they must be time-consuming or interfere with normal routines or with occupational or social functioning, and usually they impair important relationships. That was certainly Barbara's situation.

True *obsessions* are recurrent, persistent, intrusive thoughts, impulses, or images that cause the patient anxiety or distress. They aren't simply excessive real-life worries. In OCD, the afflicted person tries to suppress these thoughts or impulses by thinking another thought, or by taking some remedial action. The most common obsessional thoughts are those of contamination—like Barbara's—or doubt (repeatedly wondering and worrying whether one has performed some act such as turning off the gas jet or locking the door).

Compulsions are repetitive behaviors the person feels driven to perform in response to the obsessional thought or impulse. A typical compulsion is handwashing or constant, repetitive checking. The compulsive act is an attempt to allay anxiety generated by the obsessive thought or impulse.

Psychoanalysts view OCD as involving defense mechanisms by which the person tries to prevent becoming aware of forbidden wishes or impulses and tries to thwart or undo the consequences of those thoughts and impulses. Barbara's obsessional thoughts about hair dye contaminating her life seemed to mask a latent and illicit wish to reactivate her liaison with Jack. To banish such unacceptable (dirty) wishes (of which she may not have been fully aware at the time), she compulsively cleansed herself and her house.

For the most part, psychotherapy hasn't succeeded in treating OCD. With the advent of the newer-generation antidepressants, OCD symptoms have been relatively easy to eradicate or modify. Whether the cause of OCD is psychogenic, biogenetic, or a combination of both (most likely it's a combination), its treatment is facilitated by medication. The symptoms can be suffocated and, often, extinguished. Some patients may stay on medication for years, while others can be weaned gradually from it.

Psychiatric symptoms may appear confusing and on the surface seem to make little sense. But sometimes they mask forbidden thoughts, wishes, impulses, fears, and regrets smoldering beneath one's level of awareness. That is, until the forbidden bursts forth with terrifying vengeance.

Just as Barbara C.'s did.

Saved by a Cup of Joe

It was a bitterly cold February morning when Phil M. walked into my office at Manhattan Hospital.

His depression began in the hospital, while he was recuperating from serious injuries that occurred on the job as a police officer. After he was medically stable and ready for discharge from the general hospital, Phil agreed to spend a few weeks as an inpatient on the hospital's community psychiatric ward. It was hoped the daily structure of the setting, combined with intense treatment, would help him regain his emotional footing.

Although Phil had done fairly well on the ward and was ready to go home, the attending psychiatrist recommended he continue with additional psychotherapy as an outpatient at the hospital's clinic.

Usually when cops were referred to the clinic for evaluation it was because they had begun acting bizarrely or were noted to be overly aggressive with civilians. In those situations the police department grew concerned about an officer's ability to continue working. Sometimes we'd see a cop who'd been involved in frequent disputes with superiors or who'd been the subject of too many civilian complaints. On the other end of the spectrum, we'd occasionally see officers who'd been involved in shootouts or hostage situations and could no longer function because of nightmares, flashbacks, and uncontrollable free-floating anxiety—the hallmarks of PTSD.

In each of these situations, a psychiatric assessment was requested by the cop's commanding officer.

In fact, these examinations were called "Fitness for Duty" evaluations.

That wasn't the case with Phil. He'd been a fine cop—no disciplinary action had ever been taken against him, and no civilian complaint was ever filed. There had never been a question about his ability to function well on the job.

That is, until the work-related injury occurred. From that point onward, Phil slipped downhill.

Having read the records, I knew a great deal about him but wanted to hear his story as only he could tell it. I'd long ago learned that reading a chart or report—even one accurately recounting a patient's history and emotional status—could not come close to hearing the story from the patient himself. There was no substitute for spending time with a patient—watching, listening, and sensing the emotional tone as a traumatic experience was recounted.

Phil was a burly, forty-year-old guy whose paunch drooped over his belt. His four-days' growth of beard was dusted with white stubble. His short hair was flecked with gray. His eyes were a deep brown with black, olive-sized pupils. His fleshy face with dark pouches beneath his eyes gave him a depleted, sleep-deprived appearance.

As he settled into the chair opposite mine, he sighed and shook his head. He set a container of coffee on the end table next to his chair.

"Look at me, Doc," he said, slouching down, oozing defeat and despair. "I've put on thirty pounds since I stopped working. Look at this belly. I'm a fat slob, and I have nothin' to do. Since I got out of the hospital, I don't sleep at all; I just sit around the house eating like an animal. The only thing I feel is pain and more pain all through my arm and hand. My wife's fed up with me, and my life's circlin' the drain. It's a big zero. I got nothin', absolutely nothin.'"

"What's going on?" I asked, seeing that clearly Phil still suffered from a formidable depression, despite having been put on Tofranil, a potent antidepressant used widely at the time. All the hallmarks of depression were there: lassitude, sadness, self-deprecation, sleeplessness, an eating disturbance, poor personal hygiene, and a paucity of self-esteem.

Was he suicidal? Would he have to be hospitalized again?

I'd seen enough patients suffering from chronic physical pain to know it could be emotionally debilitating. Even devastating. Unremitting pain could drive someone to a level of misery so profound, life no longer seemed worth living. It could literally push someone to contemplate or even commit suicide.

"Hey, Doc, you look like a regular kinda guy, so I can talk here, right? I mean, I'm not psycho, am I?"

"Nah, you're not crazy. You've been through a hell of a lot. That's what I'm here for. Let's talk."

He nodded, paused, and sighed again. He peered at me through wet, bleary eyes. His brow furrowed. "I been a cop for sixteen years. I loved the job and I love this city," he said in a warbling voice. The beginnings of tears shivered on his lower eyelids. He looked away and rubbed his eyes.

"Now I can't work and we gotta move because of my condition. I can't take the cold. It makes my arm ache like a son of a bitch. We're goin' to Florida. What the hell am I gonna do down there?"

"Tell me what happened to your arm."

"It's a long story, Doc. You really wanna hear it?"

"Yes, I do," I said with a nod.

"Jesus, I'm so goddamned angry," he muttered.

"Who're you angry at?"

"The whole goddamned world."

"What's got you feeling this way?"

"I can't work. There's nothing left for me."

"C'mon, Phil. Tell me about it."

His lower lip trembled as he fought for control. Phil was the kind of guy who'd feel emasculated if he cried in front of another man. But the tears brimming on his lower eyelids were about to cascade down his face.

"It was last October." He swallowed hard. "Me and my partner were on patrol, the graveyard shift—midnight till eight. We were workin' out of the Oh-Nine—the Ninth Precinct to a civilian— me and Tom, my partner for the last five years."

He paused, staring vacantly, as though his attention had drifted away.

I waited, wondering if he was reliving that night in his mind.

He suddenly looked up as though he'd recovered his train of thought. "I was driving. Tom was in the passenger seat. We're cruising around the East Village. There'd been some protests about God-knows-what, and there were a few street disturbances. It wasn't a big thing, but we were making extra patrols, keepin' our eyes open.

"So this particular night, we stop at a deli to get some coffee— no doughnuts," he added with a hint of a grin, "and get back in the car. We're drivin' around when we get a radio call about a fire in a clothing store on East Seventh Street, right near Tompkins Square Park."

Phil reached for the coffee container, took a sip, and set it down on the side table. His hand was shaking.

"We were right around the corner," he said. His voice cracked. He coughed, brought up phlegm, swallowed hard, and then licked his lips. "So we get there before engine twenty-eight. Sure enough, we can see there's a small fire inside the place. It looked like maybe a carton's on fire, and it's pretty much contained, but it might spread. So Tom gets outta the car to get a better look, and I'm sittin' behind the wheel with the motor runnin'."

Phil leaned forward and set his elbows on his thighs. His hands were clasped so tightly, his knuckles made a cracking sound.

"I'm sittin' there, thinkin' the fire truck should get there any minute and everything's gonna be taken care of. You know, a small fire, they'll put it out in no time. My coffee's on the dash. So I reach for it, take a sip, and put the container back," he said, glancing at the container on the end table. "And as I'm leanin' back in the seat, somethin' happens. It's so quick, it's like . . ." He paused briefly as his lips trembled. "I don't know, it's like a blow-out—everything shatters."

Phil's eyes narrowed. His face seemed to tighten.

"The windshield pops and there's a spiderweb on the glass, and at that second I feel like I'm bein' kicked by a mule. I'm slammed back against the seat. Something hits me in the right armpit. It feels like I got body slammed."

Phil's entire body flinched, though he seemed unaware of it.

"I try callin' for Tom, but the words stick in my throat. The next thing I know, I'm lyin' across the seat and I'm covered in blood. I reach for the radio, but the receiver falls onto the floor, and I can't get to it."

Phil's trembling right hand shot out, as though he were in that patrol car. There was no doubt he was reliving the incident right there in the office.

"I'm feelin' around for the thing—my hand's slappin' around in the dark on the floor—but I can't find it. I don't know what's goin' on. My head's spinnin' and I'm startin' to get dizzy. I'm bleedin' all over the place, and I feel nothin' in my right arm. It goes numb, like it's not even there.

"Then everythin' goes white on me, and it's all swirlin'. I knew I musta been shot, but I'm confused; and I'm lyin' on the seat like a sack of potatoes. And Christ on a bike, there's blood everywhere."

Phil shuddered.

"I dunno what happened next, but I hear Tom open the driver's side door, and he shoves me, tryin' to get me over to the passenger side.

"He finally gets me out from behind the wheel and jumps in, and the next thing I remember, the siren starts up. Then there're poppin' sounds and bullets're hittin' the patrol car. Pop, pop, pop." Phil flinched. His shoulders hunched and the blood drained from his face. "Bullets're comin' through the window; they're slammin' into the hood, bouncin' off the roof, hittin' everywhere. Glass is flyin' and everything's spinnin', and I don't know what the hell's goin' on.

"Tom throws the car into drive, but the damned thing stalls and bullets're hittin' everywhere. Tom tries again and again, but the engine's just whirrin'. By this time I'm on the floor and pretty much out of it.

"Finally, Tom gets the car started and I'm passin' out from blood loss—maybe from panic. I don't know." He paused, and then looked up at me. "Ya know what, Doc? I don't even remember the ride to the hospital. All I remember is the siren and Tom's yellin' somethin', but it's all hazy.

"The next thing I know, there're lights and doctors everywhere. Things're spinnin' outta control. I'm in the ER, and they're rushin' me into surgery. It's a bullet wound in the armpit. It nicked an artery and I'm bleedin' out."

Phil eyed the container of coffee. He shook his head again.

"And I learn later that a bunch of nerves got ripped apart—something called the brachial plexus. Damned thing controls everything from the armpit to the fingertips."

Phil's face was moist; a streak of sweat trickled down from his right sideburn. His face was bone white. He picked up the coffee container. It trembled so badly in his hand, he set it back on the table.

"Anyway, Doc, I had surgery. I ended up havin' four surgeries. And no matter what I do—surgery, hot packs, ice, physical therapy—my right arm isn't worth a damn. I can't move it fast.

There's just too much pain. I can lift it maybe this high, no more, and it hurts like hell when I do." Phil slowly raised his arm chest high, wincing in the process. "The worst thing's the pain—I don't know how to describe it. It's a combination of burning and, believe it or not, ice-cold feelings. It's like someone's holding my arm against a hot iron and at the same time pressing ice on it to the point where the ice-cold feeling sears into me. It runs from my shoulder down to my fingertips. And it's always there.

"The thing is . . . I can't work no more. No doc's gonna give me medical clearance, not with this thing." Phil slowly raised his right arm, using his left hand to support it. "I can't even do god-damned desk duty. I can't write or use a computer. Nowadays they make you put in your retirement papers when the docs classify you as permanently disabled. And that's what I am . . . per-manently disabled."

He rubbed his right hand with his left, grimacing in pain.

"It's burnin' right now, and in cold weather like today, the pain's unbearable. So . . . we're movin' to Florida."

I nodded, knowing there was little I could say to lessen Phil's despair. He wasn't the kind of guy who would be helped by uncovering deeply buried conflicts or making penetrating psychological interpretations. Besides, what was there to unearth? The cause of his anguish was painfully obvious. Maybe he'd eventually adapt to the new reality of his life.

But he didn't seem ready to make any psychological changes. I wasn't certain supportive counseling would help. Maybe, in time, but not at that moment.

"Bein' a cop's the only job I ever had. I don't know anythin' else. I got nowhere to go, 'cept Florida, where I'll live with the old people."

He hunched over. I almost had the feeling he would fall from the chair.

He paused, straightened up, and looked at me.

"Then ya know what happens?" he muttered. "Get this. A

month later they catch the bastard who shot me. He was nabbed after he killed an old lady he was muggin' in the neighborhood.

"So they interrogate him—sweat the son of a bitch. He admits settin' the fire in that store. Bastard was waitin' for firefighters and cops to show up so he could ambush 'em from a rooftop across the street. That's where he was when he got a bead on me.

"And now I can't sleep at night. I dream about it, terrible dreams. God-awful shit, like it's happenin' again and again. The whole thing—seein' the fire, sittin' in the car when the window shatters, and the blast of that impact. And then I hear the bullets slammin' into the car like we're in a war zone.

"The dream's so bad, I jump outta bed, sweatin' and shakin'. And my heart feels like it's gonna pump through my chest. After that I can't sleep, not for a minute. I pace the house, look out the windows, raid the refrigerator, and sit up all night just thinkin' about that night and what it did to me. It never leaves me, not for a second. It's there all day, every day . . . It never leaves, just like the pain.

"If I hear a siren or see a fire truck, a cop, or a firefighter, I feel like jumpin' outta my skin. It all comes back to me—not like it happened back then, but like it's happenin' again right now.

"I can't watch TV because whenever someone gets shot, I feel nervous. No, it's more than that; it's like an alarm goes off inside, and it all comes back to me. I'm in the front seat of that patrol car, and the bullets are flyin' and I'm bleedin' and half-dead and Tom's tryin' to get the engine started and the glass is poppin' all over the place and the room spins and I feel like I'm gonna faint."

Sweat poured from Phil's hairline. The blood had drained completely from his face. He sat there trembling, his lower lip quivering.

It was clear Phil had developed PTSD on top of a clinical depression.

His eyes roamed around the office before settling on the far wall. For a moment there was complete silence. He seemed to be trying to calm himself.

Finally, the silence ended.

"Ya know what else is goin' on, Doc? That motor inside me . . . it never stops. It runs all day, like I'm wired up. Ya know what I feel like . . . ? I feel . . ." He paused, closed his eyes once more, shook his head, opened his eyes, and stared at me. "I feel raw, like a nerve dipped in the ocean."

Rubbing his right arm, he grimaced.

"And the pain . . . it takes me back to that night, and I relive it, every second of what happened. Asleep or awake, day or night, I can't get away from it.

"And what do I have now, Doc? Absolutely nothin'," he said with a catch in his throat. "No job and no prospects. I can't even bag groceries at Publix or Winn-Dixie down there in Pompano Beach, where we're movin'. Hell, I can't even drive a car unless I use my left hand on the wheel.

"And here's the strangest thing, Doc. The bastard who shot me? Get this. He had a four-power scope on that rifle. He had me in the crosshairs—dead in his sights.

"When they interrogated him, bastard said he wanted to blow my heart out. The crosshairs were right on my ticker. But when I leaned back after setting the coffee on the dashboard, the bullet got me in the right armpit, not the heart."

Phil's hands went to his face; he rubbed his cheeks. Then he peered at me.

"If I hadn't been leanin' back when he pulled the trigger, he'd a got me in the heart. Believe it or not, that coffee saved my life—I was saved by a cup of joe."

It was all so sad. My jaw clenched and a thick, constricting feeling formed in my throat.

The room was deathly quiet. Phil stared off into space.

"When are you moving?" I finally asked.

"Next month. We're renting for a while, till we find a place to buy."

"You'll probably have less pain in the warm weather," I offered.

"Maybe. But I'll be retired, livin' with the snowbirds, the retirees. I'll be doin' nothin, just gettin' old."

"What about retraining . . . something where you won't have to use your right arm so much?" As I spoke, the words sounded hollow, unrealistic.

"What am I gonna retrain for?"

Phil was right. What could I say?

I thought about contacting the Broward County Medical Society and asking for a referral to a psychiatrist or psychologist for Phil. I told Phil I would make a telephone call and do my best to find someone he could see in Florida.

"Do you think it'll help?"

"I do. I think you can be helped to make an adjustment to life there."

Yes, if Phil could be referred to someone, there was a chance for hope.

But something struck me at that moment: *my* hopes and *his* hopes didn't necessarily coincide.

The best hope might simply be tincture of time: maybe over the course of a few months, living in warmer weather, Phil would have less pain. Maybe he'd be able to regroup psychologically and go on with some kind of reasonable life.

And maybe with the move—a change of location, away from New York City with its crowds and sirens and fire trucks—things would be better for Phil. Maybe the horror of that night would fade.

But how could anyone know?

Phil raised his head and looked at me.

"So now it's gonna be Florida . . ."

His eyes were watery again.

"Hey, Doc, you know what they call Florida?"

"What?"

"God's waiting room."

He reached for that container of coffee.

Afterword

Phil and his wife moved to Florida. I never learned if he sought treatment or how he fared after my brief contact with him.

It was clear he'd become profoundly depressed and developed the classic signs and symptoms of post-traumatic stress disorder. Both forms of pathology resulted from what happened that fateful night.

Comparing Phil's situation with that of Nathan B. (the king of the Puerto Ricans) demonstrates similarities *and* differences in their reactions to life-altering events. Both men developed PTSD, and both were depressed. Their depressions were related to no longer being able to work because of a physical injury. While their PTSD presented with similar signs and symptoms, each arrived at his pathology by a completely different pathway.

Nathan's pathology was delayed, taking *forty years* to find expression, doing so only when work no longer soaked up his mental and emotional energies. When work no longer inoculated him, his life fell apart. He became psychotic, along with having developed PTSD.

In contrast, Phil experienced the onset of PTSD *immediately* after the night he was shot. From a technical diagnostic standpoint, one must wait a full thirty days after the traumatic incident before diagnosing someone with PTSD. Before that month has elapsed, the person is viewed as suffering from acute stress disorder. (For more about PTSD, see the glossary.) Nonetheless, the onset of each man's illness was vastly different.

Another important difference between Nathan and Phil was the *duration of time* over which the traumatic events occurred.

While both men's experiences were catastrophic threats to life and limb, Nathan's illness was the result of *years* living amid the horrors of Auschwitz. In contrast to Nathan's, the stressor evoking Phil's PTSD took place in a *split second*, when a bullet penetrated the police cruiser's window. (The same could be said of Patricia A. in "Baptism by Fire" who, while grieving her dead husband, suffered the trauma of a *momentary glance* at his broken neck in the casket, resulting in PTSD.)

Another crucial difference between Nathan's disorder and Phil's involved their physical injuries. Phil's wound left him in constant pain, with alternating periods of numbness and coldness in his arm due to extensive nerve damage. Each and every sensation—minute by minute—was a potent reminder of the night he nearly lost his life. But Nathan's physical condition was far different: once his back healed, he resumed working, albeit on smaller jobs, and returned to his earlier psychologic equilibrium, thus relegating the horrors of his past to the farthest recesses of his mind.

Part of Nathan's illness involved his developing delusions of grandeur—in his mind, he'd become king of the Puerto Ricans and thought he could save these downtrodden people from disaster. In fantasy, he was undoing his horrific past and remaking his world into one where instead of being a helpless victim, he was a hero. Phil, on the other hand, was not psychotic. He simply succumbed to his nighttime dreams, his flashbacks, and his need to avoid anything reminiscent of the traumatic night when he nearly lost his life.

Nathan's injury tore away his protective shell, left him feeling helpless, and thrust him back to an earlier trauma *unrelated* to the injury he sustained at work. But Phil's wound was a critical component of the incident bringing on PTSD.

Of vital importance is this singular fact: both men shared the *same* diagnoses yet presented in vastly *different* ways. The precipitating events were completely unalike, as was each man's ability to adapt to the harsh reality of his changed life circumstances.

In psychiatry, even when diagnoses are precisely the same, no two patients are truly alike.

Each person is unique, with a distinct causative event, a dissimilar onset of illness, a variable duration and depth of pathology, and an individually determined resolution, if one is to be had.

Each patient has a different and compelling story to tell.

In psychiatry, a diagnostic label may be of little value unless the psychiatrist appreciates the circumstances behind the presenting illness.

When a Patient Knows More Than the Doctor

One year out of my residency, when I was an attending psychiatrist at the hospital, my duties involved supervising residents working on the wards and teaching occasional classes. Because many residents were stricken by the flu, I was covering the liaison service, when, on a bitterly cold night, I received a call from a surgeon.

"I have a thirty-nine-year-old woman here who's physically stable," he explained. "She was brought in a few nights ago after jumping in front of a subway train. She lost her left leg and had an above-the-knee amputation. She's ready for transfer to the rehab unit, but while she's medically cleared, I feel she should be psychiatrically evaluated. After all, she made a serious suicide attempt."

Walking toward the general hospital, I wondered what could drive someone to jump in front of an oncoming train. Losing a parent? A lover? A friend? A job? Learning you've contracted a terminal disease?

Willie Mae E. was a thin woman who shared a room with five other women. She was dozing in bed when I entered the room.

She was no longer receiving IV fluids. The amputation stump was neatly bandaged.

She awoke as I approached and peered at me with narrowed eyes. I introduced myself and pulled a chair up to her bedside. The moment I told her my name, she turned away. It was clear she was mistrustful. Her hair was unruly. Although the aides had sponge-bathed her after surgery, I got the distinct impression she hadn't been properly caring for herself for quite a while. Everything about her—her disheveled look, her suspiciousness, her desperate act of self-destruction—made me suspect she suffered from schizophrenia.

The surgical chart noted she'd had "multiple psychiatric hospitalizations," although the records from those hospital stays weren't available on the surgical ward. According to the chart, she had no recollection of the psychiatric facilities to which she'd been admitted over the years.

Those were precomputer days, so I wasn't able to easily access her previous records, even from our own facility, but I had a hunch she'd been hospitalized on one of our psychiatric wards and reminded myself to search for her records when I returned to the psychiatric building.

"How're you feeling?" I asked.

"Could be better," she said, still looking away.

"What's wrong?"

She turned to me. "My leg, for one thing. It hurts like hell. Especially the toes," she said, pointing toward her missing leg.

She was describing phantom limb pain, commonly experienced after an amputation. Even though the limb was gone, its presence was still embedded in her brain's representational view of her body. Phantom limb pain occurred in virtually every amputee and could last for months, years, or even a lifetime.

"Did the surgeons explain what the pain is?"

"Yup . . ."

"And how do you feel emotionally?"

"I'd be much better if they'd stop talking to me . . ."

"If who would stop talking to you?"

"The voices."

"You mean voices in your head?"

"They're not in my head. They're everywhere."

"Are they in this room?"

"Yup. And they don't shut up."

"What are they saying to you?"

"They tell me to do things."

My antennae shot skyward.

"What kinds of things?" I asked.

"Oh . . . get up . . . go to the bathroom. Turn on the TV. Eat now. Go to sleep."

She was describing *command hallucinations*—the most dangerous of all auditory hallucinations. Those voices—products of her chaotically disturbed mind—could compel her to do anything, and despite attempts to resist them, the directives held sway over her free will. A person experiencing command hallucinations would eventually succumb to the dictates of those inner demons—even if they ordered her to jump in front of a subway train. The surgical resident's caution about her had been right on the money.

"Ms. E . . . you said *voices*. How many are there?"

"Two . . ."

"Are they people you know?"

"No. Strangers," she mumbled, looking away.

"Men, women . . . ?"

"A man and a woman."

"Do they talk to each other or only to you?"

"Both."

"What do they say?"

She cocked her head and appeared to be listening intently. No doubt she was hearing them at that moment.

It was important to determine if they talked *to* her or *about*

her. Often *alcoholic hallucinosis* (hallucinations caused by withdrawal from excessive alcohol) involved voices talking to each
other *about* the person, while schizophrenia usually presented
with voices talking *to* the person, though there could be a mixture of both.

She said nothing; she was obviously listening intently.

"What are the voices saying?"

"What do they say?" she replied, again looking at me. "'Oh . . .
look at her . . . She's going to the bathroom now' . . . or . . . 'Do
you hear what she's thinking . . . the evil things she thinks? She
deserves to die.'"

"When they talk directly to *you*, what do they say?"

"Like I said, they tell me to do things."

"What kinds of things?"

She shook her head.

"Do they tell you to do bad things?"

"Sometimes," she whispered.

"Like what?"

She remained silent, stared vacuously into space. It was obvious: she was lost in her inner mental torment, floating in a haze
of inner preoccupation. No doubt she was chronically afflicted
with the hallmarks of schizophrenia.

"Did the voices tell you to jump in front of the train?"

She closed her eyes and nodded.

"What did they say, exactly?"

"Do it. Jump now." Tears streamed from her closed eyes.

An eerie feeling pervaded me. While despair may have been
part of what drove her to jump, the real impetus was a command
from one or both voices—dictates of self-destruction coming
from the deepest recesses of her mind. Whether they were products of aberrant brain chemistry or emotional issues was irrelevant. They'd commanded her, and she'd obeyed. It was imperative
to save her from her own destructive impulses.

She opened her eyes. While they were vacant-looking only minutes earlier, now they were focused on something. She tilted her head as though listening intently.

"Are they talking to you right now . . . the voices?"

She nodded her head.

"What are they saying?"

"They're telling me not to listen to you."

She was hallucinating right there on the surgical ward. She was psychotic—had lost touch with reality, was living in a world of her own sick creation, hearing the commands of imaginary voices.

There was no way she could be discharged. It would be a death sentence.

I made arrangements for her to be transferred to the psychiatric hospital. Rehab could send a physical therapist to work with her on the third-floor women's ward.

Later that evening I located her psychiatric records.

Willie Mae E. had been hospitalized at our facility many times over the decades. The records—six inches thick—made it clear: for years she'd suffered from paranoid schizophrenia. After brief stays and having been placed on antipsychotic medication, she'd recovered her sanity and was discharged.

She'd also made the rounds to other local hospitals: Bellevue, Franklin Hospital, Roosevelt Hospital, Midtown East Hospital, and Beekman Downtown Hospital. She was known in virtually every Manhattan psychiatric facility.

In each instance the story was nearly identical: After discontinuing her medication, she would present with a resurgence of auditory hallucinations. The voices would return and command her to harm herself.

After each admission and discharge, she was assigned to an

outpatient clinic for once-monthly follow-up. So long as she visited the clinic for periodic medication adjustments, she led a reasonably normal life and worked in a commercial laundry.

But for reasons known only to her, she would stop taking her medication. Decompensation quickly followed. The voices would return with their insistent commands, and invariably, she would end up in a hospital.

It was a revolving door. A common scenario for many chronically psychotic patients.

The medication was her lifeline to relative normality. The good news in this otherwise depressing scenario was simple: despite the recurring nature of her illness, when she stopped her medication, she retained enough insight to find her way to the nearest psychiatric facility for help.

But this time she'd fallen victim to the voices.

About six months later I received a telephone call from a man who identified himself as Max Hoffman. "Doctor," he said, "I'd like to come see you. It's about your former patient Willie Mae E. Do you remember her?"

"Yes. I treated her a while ago . . . briefly. I haven't seen her since she was discharged."

"I'd like to talk with you about her."

Feeling a bit wary, I asked, "What's your relationship to her?"

"I'm her attorney. I represent her in a personal injury lawsuit."

"How'd you get my name?"

"From the hospital records. You were the psychiatrist who saw her after she jumped in front of the train. And you treated her on the ward."

"Yes, I did. Tell me, who's she suing . . . and what for?"

"I'll tell you more about it when we meet."

"Is she suing Manhattan Hospital?"

"Not at all. She received excellent treatment at your facility."
My curiosity was piqued.

Max Hoffman was a burly man in his early sixties. He looked
like he'd once been an NFL linebacker. He had broad shoulders, a
massive chest, a thick neck, and a flattened nose, and was steep-
jawed. He looked exactly how I expected a pugnacious personal
injury attorney to appear.

After a brief introduction, he began. "Let me tell you why I'm
here."

I leaned back in my chair, ready to listen.

"As you know, Ms. E. lost a leg after she jumped into the path
of an oncoming train."

"Yes, I remember her well," I said, recalling having trudged
to the surgical ward on that cold winter night. I wondered if she
was suing the Transit Authority. Over the months, I'd not only
thought of Willie Mae, but wondered about the poor motorman
driving that train. What did he experience as he approached the
station? He must have seen this figure, perhaps backlit by the station lights, leaping into the path of the train he knew he couldn't
stop in time. No doubt he'd frantically jammed on the brakes.
What were his thoughts at the moment of impact? And how did
he feel when he saw Willie Mae being extricated from the tracks?
Has he been consumed by irrational feelings of guilt? Could he
ever work as a motorman again?

I was reminded that suicide, or a suicide attempt, almost
always leaves more than one victim in its wake.

Hoffman said, "I'm sure you recall Willie Mae was out of the
hospital two weeks after you put her back on Risperdal—the
medication she'd stopped taking before she jumped in front of
that train."

"Yes, I remember."

"Well, she's suing Midtown East Hospital."

"Midtown East?" I said, thinking I'd misheard him. "She was at *Manhattan* Hospital."

"I'll get to that very soon." Hoffman reached into his briefcase and removed a sheaf of papers. "You saw her about six months ago, right?"

"Yes, but I can't violate her confidentiality by talking about her."

"Ordinarily that's true. But when a patient files a medical malpractice lawsuit—as Willie Mae has—she forfeits the right to confidentiality since her medical treatment is called into question. It becomes public record, just as a trial is public record. So there's no confidentiality here."

I nodded. It was my second interface with forensic psychiatry, the other being my testimony at Patricia A.'s hearing some years earlier.

"Okay, so there's no confidentiality," I said. "Now, what does this have to do with Midtown East Hospital and me?"

Hoffman smiled and nodded. "Okay, let's get to the heart of the matter." He paused for a moment and then continued. "Are you aware that only a half hour before she jumped in front of that subway train, Willie Mae was seen by a psychiatrist at Midtown East?"

That was a startling revelation.

"I didn't know that." My pulse quickened.

"I have the hospital records right here. And I have a transcript of the deposition testimony of the psychiatrist who evaluated her that night—a half hour before she jumped. He's Dr. Richard Cantwell. Do you know him?"

"No."

"Good. Because if you did, I couldn't use you as a witness. Let me tell you what happened. Then I'll leave the records with you and you can decide if you want to be involved in the case."

Hoffman set the papers on the end table beside his chair.

"The night she jumped," Hoffman said, "Willie Mae was hearing voices telling her to kill herself. She'd stopped taking her medication a week earlier. The night she went to the Midtown East emergency room, she was very scared. She was still sane enough to try to disobey the voices. So she went to Midtown East for help. As you probably know, this was one of *many* times when this kind of thing happened with her."

I nodded.

"She told Cantwell the voices were telling her to *kill herself.*"

I wondered why she hadn't been committed to Midtown East at that moment.

"Cantwell had her previous charts from Midtown East since she'd gone there many times. So he knew her history, or rather, had her history available to him. She told him she'd stopped taking the Risperdal a week earlier because it made her tired.

"Mind you, this is all in the hospital records—every bit of it—and Cantwell confirmed this in his deposition testimony.

"Willie Mae wanted to be admitted, but Cantwell refused. He told her he'd prescribe another medication with fewer side effects."

What made Cantwell decide not to admit her?

"Willie Mae knew it would take time for the new medication to build up in her system. She told Cantwell she'd only feel safe in the hospital."

Hoffman peered at me, apparently trying to determine the story's impact on me. I tried keeping my facial expression neutral, but disbelief seeped through me.

Willie Mae's self-assessment had been completely on target. By the time she saw Cantwell, the Risperdal had cleared her system. It would take at *least* a week before a new medication would reach a therapeutic level. During that week, she would remain dangerously psychotic.

"Well," Hoffman went on, "to make this even more unbelievable, Cantwell told her to go home and take time off from work.

She told Cantwell she was afraid she'd hurt herself before the medication kicked in. But he wrote the prescription anyway and advised her to take the first dose right there in the ER, to use the water fountain.

"Then, pathetically, Willie Mae *begged* Cantwell to admit her for the night. She couldn't trust herself to make it back home safely. Cantwell told her to take the medication and go home.

"She was so desperate to stay," Hoffman said, "she told Cantwell she didn't have the money to get home. So guess what?"

Hoffman paused.

I waited, wondering what would come next.

"This son of a bitch reached into his pocket and handed her a *subway token*. And he told her to take the train home."

A psychiatrist hears this story from a totally decompensated patient with a long history of hospital admissions. She's hearing voices—command hallucinations—telling her to kill herself and begs to be admitted to the hospital. But he's so intent on sending her home, he hands her a subway token? Unbelievable.

"So she leaves Midtown East," Hoffman said. "She makes her way to the subway station, uses the token Cantwell gave her, stands on the platform, and as the train pulls in, she jumps. And, of course, she loses a leg."

Hoffman paused. His eyebrows arched.

"Are you asking if I'm willing to be a witness in this case?"

"Yes. I need an expert witness. But let me ask you something. Are you familiar with what's needed for a plaintiff to prevail in a medical malpractice case?"

"Not at all."

"Let me explain," Hoffman said, moving his bulk forward in the chair. "A medical malpractice case is, of course, a civil matter. But it's different from other personal injury cases."

"How?"

"In a med-mal case, the plaintiff must show by a preponderance

of evidence that the physician or hospital—the defendant—
departed from standard medical or psychiatric practice while
treating the patient. The issue of departure from standard practice is crucial for a plaintiff to prevail.

"It's not just a matter of a bad result . . . let's say, a patient
who dies on the table during an operation. That's a bad result.
But to prevail in a med-mal suit, the plaintiff must show the surgeon *departed* from standard surgical practice—let's say, he was
careless and cut an artery, didn't notice it, sewed the patient back
up, and the patient bled to death. Or maybe, the surgeon left a
sponge in the patient's abdominal cavity."

Hoffman paused. "Are you with me so far?"

"Yes, I get it. There must be a departure of some kind."

"Right. That departure constitutes negligence. In addition, the
plaintiff must show by a preponderance of evidence that the doctor's departure was the *proximate* cause of damages suffered by
the patient.

"In the law, the concept of proximate cause is vitally important," Hoffman said. "It means the physician's departure must
be the *direct cause* of whatever damages the patient sustained. If
I open you up and sever an artery but it manages to close itself
off and heal, and then you die a week later from, let's say, a ruptured appendix, there's no proximate cause between my departure and your death. So there's no case to be brought against
me. Got it?"

I nodded.

"Now, there's another difference between a medical malpractice case and an ordinary personal injury case. In a personal
injury matter—let's say, an automobile accident where a driver
is speeding, hits a pedestrian, and breaks the guy's legs—the jury
can decide for the plaintiff by a simple majority, meaning only
four of the six jurors need to find in favor of the plaintiff.

"But in a med-mal case, the burden of proof is higher. The

jury must decide *unanimously*—all six jurors must agree—there was a departure from standard and accepted medical practice.

"*And* they must unanimously agree the departure was *directly and causally related* to the injury suffered by the plaintiff. In other words, my severing your artery must lead directly to your injury or death."

"You're painting a very clear picture," I said.

Hoffman's eyes bored into me. "Do you think Cantwell departed from standard and accepted psychiatric practice by sending Willie Mae home that night?"

"It seems that way. I'd have to look at the records to be certain."

"Understood," Hoffman said. "I'll leave them with you. If, after reviewing the records along with what I've told you, you're willing to be an expert witness, we can talk about it. I'll certainly compensate you for time spent reviewing the records."

Ten months later I sat in a chair on the witness stand in a courtroom at 60 Centre Street, New York's Supreme Court in Lower Manhattan. The room had high ceilings, casement windows, massive art deco chandeliers, and old wooden gallery benches. The jury box was to the left of the witness stand.

The Honorable A. J. Bronz—a bald, bespectacled wisp of a man—presided at the bench, a massive mahogany desk elevated a few feet above the witness chair.

Willie Mae E. was at the plaintiff's table beside Hoffman. She appeared subdued and was dressed in a white blouse with a simple knee-length gray skirt, which allowed her right-leg prosthesis to be seen.

The jurors were a group of conscripted citizens—six regular jurors and three alternate jury members—sitting in two rows off to my left. They ranged in age from their midtwenties to their sixties.

I was called as the last witness for the plaintiff's case.

Hoffman's voice boomed through the courtroom as he took me through my qualifications—my education, training, and psychiatric experience. He then turned to the judge and said, "Your Honor, based on his training, credentials, and experience, I ask that the witness be qualified as an expert in psychiatry."

"He is so qualified," ruled the judge. "As such, he may render an opinion in the field of psychiatry."

Hoffman then asked me about consulting with Willie Mae E. on the surgical ward the night I was called to see her. He questioned me about my evaluation of her, the voices she heard and their commands, and my decision to have her admitted to the psychiatric hospital. He then asked about her recovery over the course of two weeks on the psychiatric ward.

Referring to hospital records, he posed questions designed to elicit her history of more than a dozen psychiatric admissions, each followed by rapid recovery after hospitalization. He asked other pointed questions, bringing out the uncontestable fact that, unlike many chronically psychotic patients, Willie Mae E. was a highly functioning person when she took her medication. She had never required long-term institutionalization.

He asked me to define and describe to the jury auditory hallucinations, concentrating on the danger of command hallucinations, such as those that had plagued Willie Mae E.

He questioned me about Willie Mae's meeting with Dr. Cantwell, who was not in court, presumably because of a personal family matter. His absence relieved me of the need to be critical of his treatment while he sat at the defense table.

Referring to the Midtown East Hospital records, Hoffman asked me to describe Dr. Cantwell's refusal to admit her to the hospital. The jurors were already familiar with this key issue, having heard Ms. E.'s own testimony and having heard Dr. Cantwell himself, whom Hoffman had subpoenaed to testify. According to Hoffman, Cantwell acknowledged having not looked at the prior records from Midtown East before examining Ms. E. However, in his testimony Cantwell insisted he'd used his best judgment about her suicidal potential during his evaluation.

Even though they knew the entire story, the jury appeared to be listening in rapt attention as I spoke.

The defense attorney, a tall, slender woman named Mary Driscoll, sat at the defense table, fixing her eyes on me as I testified. It was unnerving. I was being scrutinized in preparation for the cross-examination to come.

I did my best to focus on Hoffman's questions. As I answered, I made brief eye contact with each juror, as Hoffman had instructed. Some heads nodded at key points of my testimony.

Hoffman came to the core issue. "Doctor," he said, approaching the witness box. "Did Dr. Cantwell's treatment of Willie Mae E. involve a departure from standard and accepted psychiatric practice?"

"Yes, it did."

"How so?"

"The patient was obviously psychotic," I began. "She couldn't tell reality from fantasy. She was hearing voices—command hallucinations—telling her to harm herself and was afraid she would obey them. She asked to be admitted to the hospital but was sent away with a subway token. A short time later she jumped in front of a subway train."

"What should the psychiatrist have done?"

"He should have assessed the patient carefully in view of her history of psychotic episodes, followed by quick recovery during short hospital stays. That history was in her chart right there, at Midtown East. He should have realized her psychotic state could lead to self-harm, since command hallucinations are very dangerous, especially when they're telling the patient to kill herself. He should have made a considered judgment about all this and admitted her to the hospital. She needed to be protected from herself."

As I spoke Ms. Driscoll's unwavering stare continued unabated. If she was trying to intimidate me, she was succeeding. Her eyes bored into me, warning that a crushing cross-examination was coming soon.

"Now, Doctor," Hoffman continued, "you've testified that Dr. Cantwell departed from standard and accepted psychiatric practice in evaluating Willie Mae E., correct?"

"Yes."

"Furthermore, Doctor, is it your opinion that this departure by Dr. Cantwell is the direct and proximate cause of Willie Mae's having jumped in front of the subway train, resulting in the loss of her leg?"

"Yes, it is. Dr. Cantwell's departure was directly and causally related to the loss of her leg. Had he admitted her to the hospital, she could not have jumped in front of the train, and there'd have been no amputation. Based on her past history, she would very likely have recovered after a brief hospitalization at Midtown East and could have gone on with her life."

"And, Doctor, has your opinion been given with a reasonable degree of medical and psychiatric certainty?"

"Yes, it has."

"Your Honor, I have no further questions for the witness at this time."

Cross-examination began after a lunch recess.

Mary Driscoll used her considerable height—she was at least five eleven, not counting her three-inch-high heels—to her advantage. She loomed over me as I sat in the witness box, a few feet from her.

"Now, Doctor," she began, "this is the second time you've appeared in court, isn't it?"

"Yes."

"The first time was in a hearing involving Patricia A. at Manhattan Hospital some years ago, correct?"

"Yes."

She'd done her homework, had "book" on me. She probably had the transcript of the hearing with her on the defense table. And she'd likely memorized it. She would listen for anything I now said that could be inconsistent with my previous testimony. The smallest deviation—no matter how slight—would be ammunition for her legal blunderbuss. My thoughts reeled to that old case, trying to recall what I'd said back then. But it was too long ago, and besides, my thoughts were spinning with Willie Mae E.'s case.

"And in the Patricia A. case, how much were you paid to testify?"

"I wasn't paid. I was an employee of the hospital. It was part of my job."

"And now, coming into court today, you're being paid by Mr. Hoffman, true?"

"Yes."

"How much?"

"Five hundred dollars an hour."

"Five hundred dollars an hour?" Her eyes widened as she feigned shock at this exorbitant sum. She glanced at the jurors to assess their reaction.

"That's five hundred an hour, Doctor?" she repeated.

"Yes."

Driscoll paused, apparently letting my acknowledgment of the fee soak into the jury's awareness. She crooked her right elbow over her left hand and held her right hand to her mouth. After shaking her head in feigned disbelief, she strode back behind the lectern.

Hoffman had prepared me for this line of questioning. He said the average fee for a physician's courtroom testimony was $500 an hour—for time spent in meeting with the attorney, for reviewing records, and for portal-to-portal time spent in court, which was usually most of a day. Hoffman advised, "Just quote an hourly fee. If you say it's seventy-five hundred for the fifteen hours you're spending, the jury will be horrified."

Driscoll moved to her next line of questioning.

"Now, Doctor, have you ever been retained by a *defense* attorney?"

"No, I haven't."

"In fact, Doctor, this is your first time in open court, isn't it?"

"Yes, other than the hearing—"

"That's a yes or no question, Doctor."

It was obvious: Driscoll would ask only *yes* or *no* questions designed to box me into monosyllabic answers. She wanted to corner me and preclude me from elaborating. She'd do her best to paint me as a hack, a highly paid gun for hire.

Hoffman had warned about this approach. "It's standard fare on cross-examination. It's called a *collateral* attack," he said. "The attorney avoids the medical issues—which in this case are devastating for the defense—and instead focuses on the witness. She'll try to discredit you, to paint you as a whore. When I can, I'll object, but be prepared for this line of questioning."

"And, in fact," Driscoll continued, "before today, you've never been hired to testify in a medical malpractice case, have you?"

Hired. A loaded word.

"No."

"And Mr. Hoffman has hired you and is paying you for your testimony, isn't he?"

"Objection, Your Honor!" Hoffman shouted as he rose to his feet. "The doctor isn't being paid for his *testimony*. He's being paid for his *time* and *expertise*."

"The objection is sustained," ruled the judge.

"*Expertise*?" Driscoll repeated, her voice rising derisively. "Isn't it true that your experience with medical malpractice is very limited?"

"Yes . . ."

"In fact, your experience in forensic psychiatry is next to none, correct?"

"This is my second case."

"Not exactly an abundance of cases, is it?"

"No."

"Now, Doctor, have *you* ever been sued for medical malpractice?"

"No, I haven't."

"Are you absolutely *certain* of that?" Driscoll's eyebrow arched with the question. She turned suddenly and strode toward the defense table, as though she were about to retrieve some papers. It was pure bluff, but the implication she was trying to convey to the jury was clear.

"Objection, Your Honor," Hoffman called. "Asked and answered. And Ms. Driscoll's making an improper inference that the witness isn't being truthful."

"The objection is sustained."

Driscoll turned from the defense table and walked back to the lectern.

"Doctor, you testified when your attorney was questioning you—"

"Objection, Your Honor," cried Hoffman. "I'm not the witness's attorney. I represent Ms. E., *not* the witness."

"I stand corrected, Your Honor," Driscoll said, glancing at the judge. She was backtracking, realizing her attempt to paint me as an advocate—a paid hack—might be coming up short.

"Doctor," she continued, "you testified when Mr. Hoffman was questioning you on direct examination that Dr. Cantwell should have assessed the patient, correct?"

"I said he should have assessed her more carefully."

"Where did you say *more* carefully, Doctor? Nowhere in your direct testimony did you use the phrase 'more carefully.'"

I thought back to Hoffman's description of another technique I'd likely encounter on cross-examination. "She'll play word games with you," he'd said. "She'll point out any misuse of a word, or any vague word you use, or a minor omission. It's an attempt to deflect the issue away from the medicine. She'll focus on little factoids and irrelevancies."

"What I mean is—"

"Listen to my question, Doctor. Where in your testimony did you say 'more carefully'? Can you tell me that?"

"I don't recall."

As Hoffman predicted, she was into playing word games. My thoughts streaked back to direct examination.

Did I say more carefully? *I don't remember.*

"Doctor, we can have the court reporter read back your testimony word for word, and I would wager we won't find that phrase . . . more carefully.'"

"I may not have used those exact words, but that's what I meant," I said. "He should have assessed her and made a determination about her psychosis based on her past history, her potential for suicide, about her judgment and—"

"Let me stop you there, Doctor . . ."

"Objection, Your Honor!" Hoffman shouted. "Ms. Driscoll's interrupting the witness. He didn't finish his answer."

"Your Honor," Driscoll countered, "this witness is talking at length. He's going far beyond the scope of my question. I simply want him to answer *my* question . . . not lecture or pontificate to the jury."

"Objection!" shouted Hoffman. "The doctor isn't 'pontificating.'"

"Enough," shot Judge Bronz, his voice caroming through the courtroom. "Ms. Driscoll, stop interrupting the witness." Turning to me he said, "And, Doctor, I know it's difficult, but please try to keep your answers responsive to the questions asked. If you feel you can't answer a question in the form it's asked, just say so, and I'll have the attorney rephrase the question. Is that clear?"

"Yes, Your Honor." My cheeks grew hot.

The judge looked up at both attorneys and said, "Now, let's proceed."

"Doctor," Driscoll said, "before we got sidetracked, you mentioned the issue of *judgment*. Do you recall that?"

"Yes."

"Isn't it true when evaluating any patient, a physician—whether a psychiatrist, surgeon, internist, or what have you—makes a judgment call about the patient?"

"Yes. Judgment always plays a part in an assessment."

I had some notion of where this line of questioning would go.

"Would you say a physician's judgment plays a significant, even *crucial* role in assessing a patient and then making a decision?"

"Yes, that's true."

"Well, then, how do you know Dr. Cantwell didn't use good judgment?"

"I don't think he weighed the consequences of his decision not to admit Ms. E. He just sent her away."

"How do you know he didn't weigh the potential consequences of his decision?"

"The results speak for themselves."

"In other words, is it your testimony that every patient who commits suicide or attempts it is the victim of a physician who didn't make a good judgment call?"

"No. I'm saying—"

"That's a *yes* or *no* question, Doctor."

"I can't answer that question with a *yes* or *no*. It's an oversimplification and it's misleading." I maintained eye contact with Driscoll, but in my peripheral vision I saw Hoffman nodding.

It felt like my blood was beginning to bubble. But that was what Driscoll wanted—she was trying to unnerve me.

Despite Hoffman's warning about the rigors of cross-examination, this was turning out to be pure torture.

Driscoll's eyebrows rose and her lips formed a thin slash across her face. She paused and flipped a few papers on the lectern. Then she grabbed a pen and drew lines through what must have been a few prepared questions. My insisting I couldn't answer *yes* or *no* must have preempted some of her loaded questions. She looked up at me with piercing blue eyes. They looked like chips of ice.

My stomach lurched. I anticipated an excruciatingly long afternoon.

A juror began coughing. It went on for nearly a minute.

"Doctor," Driscoll said, "are there people walking around New York City who're hearing voices? People having auditory hallucinations?"

"I'm sure there are."

"Do some of them hear voices telling them to kill themselves?"

"Maybe so."

"In a city of eight million people, isn't it a good bet there are at least ten people hearing command hallucinations with voices telling them to kill themselves?"

"I really can't say."

God only knows where this line of questioning is going.

"I'm asking you to assume there are ten such people out there. Do they all jump in front of subway trains?"

"Objection, Your Honor," Hoffman called. "Irrelevant. We're talking about my client, Willie Mae E., not about some hypothetical ten people. I'm asking the court to direct Ms. Driscoll to stick to the facts of this case."

"The objection is sustained."

Driscoll's face blanched.

She would have to find another way to slant the facts of the case.

"Doctor," she went on, "does every patient who hears voices try to commit suicide?"

"No. Ms. E. certainly didn't want to commit—"

"Objection!" shouted Driscoll, looking at the judge. "The doctor is going beyond the bounds of the question. Please admonish him, Your Honor."

"Doctor," Bronz said softly, "just answer the question with a *yes* or *no* if it's put to you in such a manner. Again, if you can't answer it in the form it's presented, just say so, and I'll have the attorney rephrase the question."

"Yes, Your Honor," I said. My face felt incendiary.

"Now, Doctor," Driscoll said, moving closer to the witness stand. "I'm going to ask you once again, and please listen to His Honor's instructions. Does every patient who hears voices try to commit suicide?"

"No."

"Now, Doctor, let's get back to your opinion about Dr. Cantwell's judgment in this case." Driscoll moved back behind the lectern. "Can you testify with reasonable medical certainty about what was inside Dr. Cantwell's mind when he evaluated Ms. E.?"

"Can I read his mind, either then or now? No, I can't."

Driscoll was definitely testing my frustration quotient. Annoyance threaded through me. The needling manner of her questioning, the contemptuous tone of her voice, her feigned effrontery, and her aggressive strut were excavating my latent combativeness. Not wanting to fall victim to my emotions, I curled my toes and clenched my stomach muscles in an attempt to quell the anger simmering within me.

Stifle the irritation. Just stick it out.

"Doctor, if you can't read Dr. Cantwell's mind, then how can you know what he was considering when he made his assessment?"

"As I said, the patient's situation and the tragic results of that evening speak for themselves."

"Now, Doctor, let me ask you about the medical and psychiatric records you were paid to review for Mr. Hoffman in preparation for your testimony today. In any of these records, was there an indication *anywhere* that before the night in question, Ms. E. *ever* attempted to harm herself?" Ms. Driscoll turned from me and faced the jury.

My mind raced through everything I'd read. Was there some reference in the records I could now cite to undermine the concession Driscoll was cornering me to make?

"Not that I can recall," I was forced to reply.

"Just to be certain you haven't forgotten or overlooked something in those records," she continued, "do you want me to ask the court for a brief recess so you can double-check?"

"That won't be necessary," I replied, trying to maintain a calm voice.

"Pardon me, Doctor," she feigned. "I didn't hear your response. Please let me know if you need time to look through the records."

Hoffman remained seated. Any objection raised could very well draw more attention to my concession than Driscoll's theatrics ever would.

"I don't need additional time. There's nothing in the records."

"Well, Doctor, since there's no indication in any record that Ms. E. ever before tried to harm herself, how can you be so certain Dr. Cantwell departed from accepted psychiatric practice?"

"Because the other records indicate quite clearly that whenever she presented with command hallucinations in the past, she was hospitalized and quickly reintegrated. She was never given that chance the night she saw Dr. Cantwell. And besides—"

"But, Doctor," Driscoll cut in.

"Objection, Your Honor!" Hoffman shouted. "Ms. Driscoll's interrupting the witness."

"Sustained. Don't interrupt the witness," admonished the judge. "Doctor, have you finished your answer to the question?"

"No, Your Honor."

"Please, proceed."

"As I was saying, in an emergency-room evaluation, you have

to probe carefully and use every resource available. If a patient presents with chest pain again and again but has never had a heart attack, it doesn't mean he's not going to have one *this* time."

There was a moment of silence.

"But, Doctor," Driscoll shot, "you had the benefit of hindsight in your evaluation. You saw Ms. E. *after* she'd jumped in front of the train, and you've based your opinion on that fact. Dr. Cantwell didn't have the advantage of hindsight."

"But she was *at* the hospital *just* before she jumped in front of the train," I said. "And *that* visit to the hospital could have prevented what *did* in fact happen. *If* a careful assessment had been made."

"A *careful assessment*? Were you present in the room when Dr. Cantwell made his assessment?"

"Of course not."

A slight twitter arose from the jury box. It was an absurd question, one that seemed to be an insult to the jury's collective intelligence.

"Then how do you know he wasn't careful?" pressed Driscoll. "You weren't there. Aren't you being a 'Monday-morning quarterback,' faulting his judgment?"

"He had an obligation to the patient. It was to consider the consequences of his actions and to make an informed judgment call. And he didn't make an *informed* judgment."

"So, Doctor, in looking at the records *after* the fact, you've come to the conclusion that Dr. Cantwell failed in his obligation to make a careful assessment of the plaintiff?"

"He gave her a subway token and told her to leave the ER."

Driscoll's eyes widened and she paused. Back at the lectern, she shuffled some papers and looked at me.

"Now, Doctor, you testified that Dr. Cantwell didn't use good judgment in evaluating the plaintiff, correct?"

"Yes."

"And we're all aware that Ms. E. was psychotic at the time, correct?"

"Yes."

"And a psychotic state means a patient loses touch with reality, right?"

"Yes."

"And very often such a person has poor judgment, correct?"

"Yes, that often happens."

"And it happened in this case? Ms. E.'s judgment was impaired?"

"Because she'd obey the voices; yes, her judgment was impaired."

"And she went to Midtown East, correct?"

"Yes."

"Aren't you saying the judgment of a psychotically hallucinating person was better than that of the psychiatrist evaluating her?"

I paused before answering the question.

It was hard to believe Ms. Driscoll had opened this door for me.

"What I'm saying is, Ms. E. knew the voices could lead her to kill herself. She'd been in this situation before that night. So my answer is *yes*; under the circumstances you just described, Ms. E.'s judgment *was* better than Dr. Cantwell's."

It was as though I'd dropped a two-ton bomb on Driscoll's head. She'd been so querulously aggressive—so carping and argumentative—in her questioning, she'd recklessly plowed down a path she'd never anticipated. She'd actually summed up the case—in an all-encompassing nutshell.

She blinked repeatedly, saying nothing. A dense silence enveloped the courtroom.

"Ms. Driscoll," the judge finally interjected. "Do you have any more questions for this witness?"

"Not at this time, Your Honor," she replied in a voice barely above a whisper.

On redirect examination, Hoffman asked a few questions for

clarification, but nothing new emerged. I answered each one, measuring my words and keeping in mind that Driscoll would come at me again on recross.

By the time Hoffman finished his redirect, I felt drained and dreaded going toe-to-toe with Driscoll once again.

She rose for recross and, to my immense relief, asked only a few perfunctory questions. Her voice lacked the aggressive vigor—the fiery energy it possessed during cross-examination. Her questions seemed lackluster, anemic, tentative. I sensed she wanted me off the stand, lest I do her case more damage.

Ten minutes later, feeling an enormous sense of liberation—and utterly spent—I passed the Corinthian columns outside the courthouse entrance and headed toward the subway station.

I looked forward to getting home and pouring myself a generous glass of wine.

Two days later Hoffman called.

"I didn't want to call until the jury came in with a verdict," he said.

I could tell from the tone of his voice that the verdict had been favorable.

"So . . . ?"

"They awarded Willie Mae two million dollars—for the loss of her leg, for her pain and suffering, and for future medical costs."

"I just hope she uses some of the money to get into treatment with a good psychiatrist."

"The defense will appeal," Hoffman said. "And the award will probably be reduced; but still, it'll settle for a substantial sum. And my office has been appointed conservator, so we'll dole the money out responsibly. Willie Mae hates going to a clinic, and she's agreed to see a psychiatrist privately."

"If her medication's supervised, there's hope for her future."

"Yes, there's hope. I called to say you did a great job. The jury found your testimony honest and credible. They were outraged that Cantwell gave her a subway token and sent a grossly psychotic patient out into the streets."

"I'm not an attorney," I said, "but I thought the case was a winner from the start."

"What makes you say that?" Hoffman asked with a smile in his voice.

"Willie Mae E. knew what would happen if she left the hospital. She knew she would try to take her own life. And she did her best to convince Cantwell her insanity could be deadly."

"Very true," said Hoffman.

"And he just wanted to get her the hell out of there so he didn't have to bother with the work involved in admitting her to the hospital."

"Absolutely, even though we couldn't say that in front of the jury."

"So, Driscoll put it very well," I said. "Willie Mae E's judgment was a helluva lot better than Cantwell's."

"To put it another way," Hoffman said, "she knew more than the shrink."

Afterword

I'll never forget Willie Mae E. for two reasons.

Her lawsuit was my first experience as an expert witness in open court; and over the years forensic psychiatry—that is, the interface of psychiatry and the law—became a significant part of my practice.

Willie Mae E., a soul bedeviled by malevolent voices rising from the depths of her disturbed mind, was so needlessly harmed by the carelessness of a fellow psychiatrist. Dr. Cantwell, like all of us at times, made a hasty, unthinking decision instead of a

carefully considered one, and because of his carelessness, a chaotically troubled patient paid a heavy price.

Over the years, when the pressures of too many patients and
too little time closed in on me—as often occurred—the image of
Willie Mae E. made me stop in my haste and reconsider.

Dr. Boris Papalini

He strode quickly past my office in the psychiatric emergency room. A doctor I'd never seen before in his midthirties, wearing green surgical scrubs and a white lab coat, he looked to be a man on a mission as he made his way to the bank of elevators at the end of the corridor.

A day later, in scrubs and a lab coat, he once again passed my office. A stethoscope dangled around his neck, a contrivance often employed by physicians to set them apart from the general population. The instrument could just as easily fit in the lab coat's pocket, but some doctors wore it to display their special status.

The following day there was a knock on my office door. There he was again, still in scrubs and a lab coat, but with the addition of a green surgical cap covering his hair. Very likely he had come from an operating room.

"May I come in?" he asked.

"Sure," I said, wondering why a surgeon would want to speak with me in the psychiatric emergency room.

He entered the office and stood in front of the desk.

My eyes sought out the name embroidered in blue stitching over the left chest pocket of his lab coat:

Dr. Boris Papalini

It seemed odd: he hadn't introduced himself upon entering the room.

"I was wondering if I could sit in on an evaluation," he asked in a refined English accent.

This was becoming more intriguing by the moment.

Here was a physician in an American hospital, speaking with an English accent, sporting a Russian-sounding first name and an Italian-sounding surname, now making a most unusual request. Why would a surgeon who'd just come from a stint in the OR want to sit in on an emergency-room psychiatric evaluation? When I'd seen him previously, I'd assumed he was making rounds on a post-op patient who'd been transferred to the psych ward. I'm sure my curiosity was evident as I stood to introduce myself.

"Dr. Boris Papalini," he said, extending his hand.

That, too, was odd: physicians meeting for the first time typically wouldn't use the prefix *Doctor* when introducing themselves. Most would simply give their first and last names. Was this simply a formality born of his being from the United Kingdom?

He sounded self-assured, very professional.

His grip was strong. His hand was warm and dry.

I waved at a chair.

He sat down as I sat behind the desk.

"What brings you here?" I asked.

"Oh, I have a patient upstairs."

"Which department are you from?" I asked.

"Neurosurgery," he said, as his eyes darted about the office and then rested on the wall behind me.

"Doing a consultation on one of the wards?"

"Yes. We have a patient on the third floor. She's been feeling rather dizzy and we're trying to figure out the problem. It seems routine."

A neurosurgical consult in a situation where one with a neurologist would seem more likely?

It just didn't sound right. I felt my pulse quicken.

"Have you ruled out TIAs?" I asked, using the standard abbreviation for transient ischemic attacks, otherwise known as ministrokes.

"Well, I'm not sure . . ."

His response sounded indefinite, vague, hesitant, and uncertain.

A pang of suspicion surged through me. It seemed I'd surprised him with so specific a medical question.

"And an angiogram was done?" I asked.

"Not yet."

"How about a cystoscopy?" I asked, referring to a urological procedure having nothing to do with TIAs or anything even vaguely neurological.

"Not yet," he said and crossed one leg over the other.

His vagueness, hesitancy, and failure to know I'd asked about a urological procedure, not a neurosurgical one, clinched it. On my Richter scale of suspicion, this guy hit a full-scale ten.

"Dr. Papalini, will you excuse me for a moment?" I asked, getting up. "There's something out at the reception area I have to attend to. I'll be right back."

"Why, certainly," he said, still sitting there, looking at ease. As I rose, I thought I noticed a slight bulge in the right-hand pocket of his lab coat.

A chill ran up my spine. The back of my neck tingled.

At the reception area, I approached the clerk. "Fran," I said, "ever hear of a Dr. Papalini on staff in the hospital?"

"Not in psychiatry," she said. "But there're hundreds of doctors in different departments. Why?"

"There's a guy in my office claiming to be Dr. Boris Papalini, a so-called neurosurgeon, but I'm more than a little suspicious."

Those were precomputer days, before you could tap a few keys and bring up the entire roster of the hospital's attending physicians, interns, residents, and ancillary staff members.

And in those days, photo ID badges weren't required to be

worn by all hospital personnel as they are today. Anyone wearing a lab coat or surgical scrubs was simply assumed to be on staff.

Fran was calling neurosurgery, but I knew I had to confront this man and his claim directly and immediately.

The security guard on duty was a huge guy—probably six four and weighing a solid two hundred forty pounds. "Ernest, would you help me check out this guy in my office?" I asked him. "Something tells me he's an imposter. I can't be sure, but he may be armed."

"Sure, Doc. Let me call for another guard."

Moments later two security guards escorted me back into the office.

"Dr. Papalini," I said, "please show me some identification."

Ernest and the other guard flanked him. He glanced at them but remained seated.

"My good man, I don't have my wallet with me," he answered, scowling. "As you can see, I'm dressed in surgical garments."

"Where do you live?"

"Not far away."

The guards moved closer, looming over him.

"Where is that, exactly?" I asked.

"On Third Avenue."

"The exact address, please."

"What is this?" he said, suddenly getting to his feet.

Both guards closed in.

He plopped back down in the chair.

"Tell me your exact address, please," I said.

"What *is* this? I'm being questioned like a common criminal."

"Where did you go to medical school?" I asked.

"Here in New York."

"Where, exactly?"

"I went to Bellevue."

"Bellevue isn't a medical school. It's a hospital."

He began stammering, obviously unprepared for the grilling.

"Where did you do your internship and residency?" I asked, my words growing pressured.

He kept stammering.

The guards were ready to pounce.

"Don't touch me!" he shouted, looking up at them, his eyes wide with fear. "Don't you *dare* touch me. I'll have my assistant tell you whatever you need to know, but don't touch me."

He stood, even as the guards closed in. His hand moved toward his right pocket—toward the bulge in his lab coat. An electric shock bolted through me. Was he reaching for a weapon?

Earnest grabbed his arm. The man didn't struggle. He leaned away from Ernest and cowered as the other guard clutched his left wrist.

Together the guards wrenched his hands behind him and bound his wrists with plastic ties. The stethoscope slid off his neck, falling to the floor.

"What are you doing?" he cried. "I need to talk with my assistant."

"What's in your pocket?" I demanded.

"I need to talk to my assistant," he repeated. "That's all I was doing. Why're you treating me this way?" His lips quivered and his eyes bulged.

"What've you got in your pocket?" Ernest growled.

"My . . . my assistant," he blubbered, on the verge of tears.

Was I hearing him correctly?

Just then the bulge in his pocket moved.

"What's in there?" I pressed.

"My assistant?"

"Your assistant?"

"Yes," he said. Tears formed in his eyes. "Please, loosen these straps. They're too tight."

The bulge moved and then began squirming.

Suddenly, a brown hamster poked its head out, looked around, and darted back inside.

I didn't know whether to laugh or shake my head in amazement. The man was obviously deluded—completely psychotic.

The following day I spoke with the attending psychiatrist on the ward to which the erstwhile Dr. Papalini had been admitted.

"His name's Jerome Smith," the psychiatrist said. "Thinks he's a great doctor, actually, a scientist on the verge of some enormous discovery. He's as delusional as can be. He shuttles through homeless shelters. When he gets some money, he finds a single-room-occupancy hotel. His record of psychiatric hospitalizations would fill an entire cabinet."

"And he was here in the hospital, masquerading as a neurosurgeon," I said.

"Yes. He's been living somewhere in the hospital and went to the laundry area, where he stole scrubs and a lab coat. There's a Dr. Papalini in Pediatrics—a new attending from Argentina. This guy got his hands on a stethoscope and was eating food from discarded hospital trays. He's been getting his jollies parading around the hospital, pretending to be a doctor. Nobody knows how many examinations he's sat in on. He may've even examined a few patients."

"And nobody suspected anything?"

"Hey, you know how it is. This place is busy as hell; no one pays attention. We probably have a thousand visitors a day coming in and out of here. There're food and flower deliveries; medical deliveries, all kinds of vendors; linen service; custodial workers; and hundreds of doctors, nurses, porters, aides, LPNs coming and going all hours of the day and night. This place is a small city. So this guy slips through the cracks in the mental health system and evades hospital security."

I couldn't help but wonder what might have happened if the ersatz Dr. Boris Papalini had remained free to roam the hospital.

Afterword

One year later, in 1989, a homeless man was arrested by the New York City police.

He'd been living secretly at Bellevue Hospital.

Police said he'd been sleeping on a cot hidden behind machinery on the hospital's twenty-second floor. The space had been used to store medical equipment. The man ate hospital food taken from discarded trays near the kitchen area, stealing lab coats and scrub suits from the laundry. He'd also managed to get his hands on workers' identification cards. He then moved freely through the twenty-five-story building, purporting to be a staff member. No one thought to stop and question him.

One night, wearing a doctor's scrubs and lab coat, he entered an office where a pregnant doctor was working alone. He raped, robbed, and murdered her before slipping out of the hospital unnoticed.

He was arrested at a nearby men's shelter after three homeless men came forward with the dead doctor's credit cards. They told police the suspect had been carrying them. The detectives recovered a fur coat belonging to the victim and charged the man with the doctor's rape and murder.

The perpetrator was not the man who'd been masquerading as Dr. Boris Papalini. Rather, he was one of the thousands of homeless and psychotic people populating the city's streets, alleys, and places like Grand Central Terminal. I couldn't help wondering what might have happened had "Boris Papalini" remained free to wander through the interstices of Manhattan Hospital.

After the 1989 incident, security at all New York City hospitals was tightened.

But still, Manhattan Hospital is a mammoth institution. You don't have to be an illusionist to go completely unnoticed—to virtually disappear—in the hospital's labyrinthine maze of corridors, closets, storerooms, and countless hidden places.

Who knows how many highly disturbed people still wander freely through various hospitals—posing as staff members or even as physicians, examining patients?

This case brings into focus another issue that has plagued modern psychiatry. It surfaced regularly during my work at every hospital or outpatient clinic with which I was ever affiliated. It's the issue of *deinstitutionalization*.

With the advent of neuroleptics (antipsychotic medications) in the 1950s, mental hospitals for long-term commitment were virtually emptied out. Medications like Thorazine and Stelazine were viewed as the single greatest advance in the history of psychiatric care, markedly improving the prognoses of institutionalized psychotic people. Many severe signs and symptoms of schizophrenia, paranoia, and other major mental disorders could be suffocated or ameliorated to the point where afflicted people no longer required long-term or lifelong commitment. These patients—formerly institutionalized for years—were discharged from hospitals. If these medications were taken properly, they enabled many patients to lead reasonably normal lives out in the world.

But there was a huge catch: the medications had to be taken every day—without fail—to effectively smother these illnesses.

The new treatment model for patients with chronic, psychotic disorders was no longer institutionalization. Rather, the regimen was ongoing visits to clinics and community mental health centers. Supervised halfway houses were established for those severely compromised patients who had no family support and who lacked the ability to fend for themselves in society. The arrangement was intended to enable these people to live relatively normal lives away from the confines of locked hospital wards.

While this new model was workable for some, it failed for many others. As soon as they stopped taking medication and no longer kept clinic appointments, they deteriorated to their former psychotic states.

As a result, many highly disturbed people began cycling through psychiatric hospitals for short-term stays. Or they flooded community mental health centers in floridly psychotic states of agitation or desuetude.

These facilities were overwhelmed by the massive influx of transient patients, many of whom had formerly been institutionalized for long-term care.

The system of health care delivery was caught in an insoluble quandary.

The Americans with Disabilities Act *mandates* that psychiatric treatment must take place in the least restrictive setting possible. While this act makes a valiant attempt to preserve patients' civil liberties, it fosters the untenable situation of repeated emergency hospitalizations in an underfunded and inadequate outpatient care system.

Many patients are seen once every two to three months at community mental health centers for medication checks lasting a matter of minutes.

As a result of sporadic and inadequate support, a number of patients revert to their former psychotic states and join the ranks of the homeless living on park benches and under bridges.

For others, a return of psychosis ushers in violent, antisocial behavior, resulting in incarceration.

According to *Psychiatric News*[6] published by the American Psychiatric Association, two million people with severe mental

---

6. *Psychiatric News* 50, no. 11, June 5, 2015.

illness cycle through America's county jails every year. This creates an enormous strain on county governments, who are required
to provide them with treatment. The budgetary costs involving
police personnel, psychiatric intervention, food, medication, and
other expenses take a huge toll on local governments.

Jerome Smith, aka Dr. Boris Papalini, was one such patient
whom the system failed. Once he stopped taking medication
and failed to keep clinic appointments, he decompensated. In his
delusional state, he wandered from one facility to another, completely out of touch with reality.

He became part of the "revolving door" system that continues
today: repeated short-term hospitalizations on psychiatric wards,
stabilization, discharge, missed clinic appointments, failure to
take medication, resurgence of madness, all funneling down a
final common pathway to rehospitalization.

This perpetual recycling of patients—in and out of hospitals—
and on-again, off-again pharmacotherapy leads inevitably to a
formidable level of deterioration in a person's mental and emotional functioning. Over a period of years, it results in a worsening of the illness, which some theorists have called *downward
drift*. It denotes the inevitable decline in a person's social and eco-
nomic status as seen in untreated or partially treated psychosis.

There are no easy answers. The discussion continues—as it
has for years—trying to balance individual civil liberties and
patients' rights with what's required to deliver effective, lasting
treatment for the good of the patient and the community.

To date the balance has not been struck.

Off the Wall

One evening in July, though I was an attending psychiatrist at Manhattan Hospital, I was covering the psychiatric emergency room because we were short-handed.

A third-year medical student was observing evaluations as part of his rotation through the psychiatry service. After each interview, we would discuss the case. This kind of on-the-job training had long been the teaching model for medical students beyond the preclinical courses of the first year.

While we were talking about the last patient we'd seen, bellowing erupted from the waiting area. Based on many previous experiences, I suspected the shouter was an agitated psychotic man, probably dragged in by the police. My suspicion was confirmed when we stepped out of the office and saw a disheveled, handcuffed man accompanied by two cops.

The officers struggled to control him as he rose from his seat, wrestled away from them, and bolted toward the exit. A brief struggle followed, during which he was subdued. They held him firmly in place while an attendant rolled a high-backed wheelchair toward them.

"I don't wanna live!" he howled.

"You gonna admit him, Doc?" one officer asked breathlessly as we approached.

"Let me talk to him," I said, trying to make eye contact with the man.

His glazed eyes were red, swollen, unfocused.

"What's his name?" I asked.

"Who knows? He's got no wallet, no ID, nothing. He's another 'John Doe.'"

"Where'd you find him?"

"In the middle of Third Avenue, trying to jump in front of traffic."

I moved closer. Three attendants were holding the man in place. I estimated he was in his thirties. I detected no odor of alcohol on his breath or track marks on his forearms, and he didn't look like the many heroin and cocaine addicts I'd seen, though without doing blood work you could never know if some chemical substance was wreaking havoc on his brain. Other than his shouting, "I don't wanna live," everything else he said was incoherent.

His hair was a mess; dark stubble covered his face. I sniffed deeply: there was no ureic odor of sweat, urine, or any other bodily effluent. Yes, he was unkempt, but something told me he wasn't some homeless denizen of the streets.

"What's going on?" I asked, doubting he'd answer intelligibly.

"Lemme go," he roared, still struggling.

Despite the cops' and attendants' efforts, they couldn't get him into the wheelchair. He again broke free, racing toward the emergency-room doors.

The attendants wrestled him to the floor. He writhed and shouted. Even with the two officers helping, the man managed to get to his knees and began crawling toward the exit. Five men struggled to hold this one man back.

"Jesus, this guy's a helluva lot stronger than he looks," grunted a guard.

"Agitation will do that," I said, knowing severe, psychotic decompensation could imbue a one-hundred-forty-pound man with Herculean power.

"Hello," I said as he was pinned to the floor.

He stared at me with empty eyes. I inhaled deeply, again trying to detect some odor that might hint at the source of his condition.

None.

"Talk to me," I said, again trying to break through to him.

He mumbled something under his breath.

"Tell me your name."

"I wanna die. I wanna die!" he screamed.

"Why? Why do you want to die?"

"I just wanna die," he cried.

"Tell us something about yourself."

"I wanna die."

"Don't you have any hope?"

"Hope is for fools."

"We'll have to admit him," I said to the cops, who were obviously relieved to have him taken off their hands.

"This guy's off the wall," said one officer.

"Off the wall, nuts, psycho, whatever," said the other cop. "He belongs in the loony bin."

John Doe was so agitated, it was impossible to do a physical examination. On the admitting sheet, I wrote, "Physical examination deferred due to patient's agitation."

The attendants finally wrestled the man into the wheelchair. The handcuffs were removed. With the aides restraining him, a straitjacket was slipped over his arms; the ends of the long sleeves were tied securely behind him. He was strapped to the chair with sturdy canvas belts. Rocking violently back and forth, shouting and cursing, he nearly toppled the contraption.

His cries resounded off the walls as the wheelchair was rolled toward the elevator. His voice receded down the corridor. Though it was muffled when the elevator doors closed, it was still audible as the elevator rose in the shaft.

I phoned the ward. "We have an agitated John Doe coming up. I'll be upstairs to oversee his admission when I get through with the paperwork."

"That was a quick decision to admit," said the medical student.

"Sometimes we have to act decisively. You try sorting things out later."

"Any idea of the diagnosis?" he asked.

"It looks like an agitated depression."

"But you can't be sure, right?"

"Right. Before we think about a diagnosis, we have to save him from himself. We'll address diagnosis and treatment after he's calmed down."

"He says he has no hope," said the student.

"That's at the core of every severe depression," I explained. "Hopelessness, feeling there's no future. It's why people kill themselves. It's a malignancy—like having cancer of the mind."

On the ward, the medical student accompanied me to the nursing station.

At the desk, I began writing John Doe's orders. His voice—by then hoarse from nonstop shouting—could be heard down the hallway. His yelling had degenerated into indecipherable gibberish. Occasionally we heard him roar, "Lemme go! I wanna die!"

Other patients—all quite disturbed—wandered past the nursing station, occasionally looking toward the single-occupancy room from which his voice came.

"What are you going to do?" asked the student.

"When he's calmed down, I'll do a physical. For the time being, he'll be in four-point restraints."

His wrists and ankles would be wrapped with soft straps and secured to the four corners of his hospital bed frame. He'd be completely immobilized to prevent him from hurting himself.

Turning to the charge nurse, Ms. Scott, I said, "When you have him securely restrained, draw bloods for a CBC with differential, a chem panel, and a tox screen. And label it *stat*."

She nodded.

"And please make sure he's well hydrated. Give him a cup of fruit juice every half hour until he's sedated."

She nodded again.

"If he refuses to drink, give me a call in the ER and I'll be up to start an IV. That'll be tough to do with someone this agitated."

"I'll see if we can get some juice into him right now," she said, and headed toward John Doe's room.

Turning to the medical student, I explained, "There's the danger of dehydration since he's agitated, sweating, and wrapped in canvas. He could overheat and go into electrolyte imbalance if we don't hydrate him."

Having already rotated through medicine and surgery, the student knew about the danger of dehydration.

"What do you think the tox screen will show?" he asked.

"I have no idea. But we have to see if some drug has done this. A reasonable guess would be phencyclidine—angel dust— but who knows? It could be anything or nothing. And the chem panel might show if it's a toxic or metabolic situation."

"Like what?"

"It could be liver toxicity, kidney failure, an electrolyte deficiency, or an infection. The CBC will show if there's an elevated white count. Can't take his temperature right now; his agitation's raised his body temp. If nothing shows up in the lab results, it could be a brain tumor. Time and a thorough workup will give us the answer.

"Meanwhile, I'm ordering an IM [intramuscular] injection of twenty-five milligrams of Thorazine to tranquilize him," I said. "It has sedative properties and he'll calm down. We don't know how long he's been this way, but I'm sure he's nearing exhaustion. I'll do a physical when he's asleep."

Looking over my shoulder, the student watched as I continued writing orders.

"I'm also writing an order for him to be walked down the hallway for a minute or two every half hour."

"Why's that?"

"So he won't overheat. It's cooler in the hall than in the room. Walking him will let the aides know if he's calming down. Before they walk him, they'll undo the four-point restraint and put him in a camisole," I said referring to the garment commonly known as a straitjacket. "In a camisole, there's little chance he'll do anything to himself."

Laced up and secured from behind, John Doe's arms would remain in the straitjacket sleeves and would cross in front of his torso. The ends of the sleeves would be tied behind him, immobilizing his arms and hands. But in a severely agitated patient, the camisole could hasten the onset of hyperthermia—a dangerous elevation of his body's temperature.

Still looking over my shoulder, the student asked, "What's 'CC' mean?"

"It's the closest form of observation," I said. "We have two levels of strict observation for someone like this. One is *CO— Constant Observation*. It means the patient's escorted everywhere, with the attendant no more than three feet away. Even if the patient goes to the bathroom, he's watched—constantly—in case he tries to hurt himself.

"But with this man, we'll use *CC*, meaning *Constant Contact*. The attendant must be *physically* touching him when the four-point restraint is discontinued. While the patient's out of bed, there can't be a single moment when the attendant doesn't have a hand on him."

"Even though he's in a straitjacket?"

"Even then."

"That should be called *Extreme Contact*," said the student.

"It *is* extreme. But it's necessary. Right now we have to protect him from himself. When he's calmer we'll do a physical, get the results of the blood tests, get his story, and come up with a treatment plan. So, for the time being, every half hour he gets some juice and a short walk in a camisole with the orderly holding on to him. There's no latitude."

Ms. Scott reappeared. "We got some juice into him, and he just got a shot of Thorazine," she said.

When the orders were written, I again checked in on John Doe. He was completely immobilized on the bed, staring at the ceiling.

The student and I headed back to the emergency room.

It was nearly eleven p.m.

The staff would soon be changing shifts. The medical student had left. For a change, the emergency room was quiet. It was one of those rare lulls I'd learned to appreciate. I would have time to nod off for a few precious moments. The red suicide phone had been quiet all evening—a rarity. A small cadre of people called regularly, threatening to kill themselves. We would try talking them down and convince them to come to the hospital. Or we'd get their addresses and send the police to their homes. But for a change, the suicide line was dormant.

There had been no telephone call from the ward, which meant the staff was able to get John Doe to drink fluids. I decided to head upstairs and check on his condition, and if he was sufficiently sedated, I'd do the physical examination.

Suddenly, the telephone let out an ear-piercing jangle.

No doubt it was the reception clerk alerting us to an ambulance or a patrol car heading for the emergency room to deliver some wildly agitated soul.

I picked up the telephone. "Yes?"

"Doctor, we need you up here on the fourth floor."

"What's up?"

"John Doe is injured."

"How did—" But I stopped myself. It didn't matter what happened. I had to get upstairs quickly.

Slamming down the receiver, I rushed from the office, raced down the corridor, and caught the waiting elevator.

On the way upstairs I weighed the possibilities: had John Doe gone into hyperthermia while in four-point restraints? Had he suffered a catastrophic cardiac event? Had he inhaled his own mucous and saliva, which could lead to aspiration pneumonia? Had his body shut down from complete exhaustion? Was he convulsing from PCP or some other chemical he'd ingested? Was he in a coma from whatever drug he might have swallowed or inhaled before being dragged to the hospital?

On the fourth floor, I headed toward the door of Ward 4-A.

My pass key slipped into the slot and the outer door opened.

Entering the ward's dayroom, I could see down the dimly lit corridor leading to the nursing station. A clot of staff members stood in a semicircle. Some patients in their hospital pajamas were wandering about; a few stood at the periphery of the arc formed by the staff. My heart tumbled in my chest as I hurried down the corridor.

Everyone stepped aside as I drew close.

Still wrapped in the straitjacket, John Doe lay crumpled on the floor.

He was unconscious. His eyes were closed and his mouth was partly open.

"His pulse is weak," said a nurse whose hand was on his neck.

Getting down on my knees, I felt his neck for the carotid pulse: sure enough, it was barely palpable. But his skin was warm and moist: not a sign of dehydration. I lifted his eyelids. His pupils were dilated, and when the dim hallway's light hit his eyes, they constricted sluggishly. I wasn't certain, but his left pupil seemed slightly smaller than the right one. A bad sign: maybe an intracerebral bleed—otherwise known as a stroke.

I pinched his cheek, but he was unresponsive. A nurse handed me a penlight. His pupils barely constricted when I pointed the light in his eyes. Yes, his pupils were definitely asymmetrical. This was bad news.

"Let's get this thing off him," I shouted as I turned him and began unfastening the straitjacket.

A nurse handed me a stethoscope, and when John Doe was free of restraints, I listened to his heart.

It sounded thready and weak, like a bird's fluttering wings.

"Call EMS!" I shouted as I began CPR, rhythmically pumping on his sternum. "Let's get him over to the medical ER, *stat.*"

My pulse ramped up in anticipation. "What happened?" I asked.

"You won't believe it," said Mr. Johnson, an experienced orderly. His voice was shaky.

"I'll believe anything," I gasped, still pumping away.

Johnson stood there, shaking his head. His chin trembled.

"An ambulance is on the way," called a nurse.

"So, what won't I believe?" I pressed.

"I got him out of bed, sat him up, and we slipped the camisole on him," Johnson said in a quivering voice. "He was very calm. This was his fourth trip down the hallway. He was heavily sedated. I held on to him very tightly because I didn't want him to fall."

"And . . . ?" A film of sweat formed on my forehead. "Did he fall?"

Johnson shook his head. "We were coming down the hallway . . . He was moving very slowly, and then . . ." Johnson gulped.

I waited, midcompression, for him to continue.

"He pulled away from me—he was very quick—and . . . and before I could grab him, he bent over, ran full speed, and bashed his head into the wall."

The silence was so dense, I heard blood rushing in my ears.

"He bashed his head into the *wall*?"

I interrupted the exchange to check John Doe's condition. His breathing was labored, irregular.

There was barely a heartbeat.

I was certain he'd impacted his skull with sufficient force to not only lose consciousness but cause a subdural or epidural hematoma to form—he was likely bleeding into his brain.

At that moment the EMTs arrived. They were quick and efficient. One guy whipped out a stethoscope and listened to John Doe's heart.

"I don't hear a thing," he said.

An Ambu-bag was slipped over John Doe's nose and mouth. One technician began squeezing the bag every few seconds—forcing air into his lungs—while the other resumed chest compressions.

Still giving CPR, they lifted him onto a gurney, wheeled him to the elevator, rode down four flights, went out through the emergency-room doors, and loaded him onto an ambulance.

He was whisked away to the general hospital.

Some hours later the complete blood count with differential, the tox screen, and the chemistry panel came back from the lab. The toxicology report was negative for illicit substances. The chem panel showed no evidence of a toxic or metabolic disorder. And there was no indication in the blood count of an infection or any other abnormality. As best could be deduced, there was no medical reason for the man's insanely agitated, suicidal state. It was purely psychological.

The next day I learned the autopsy results: John Doe died from an epidural hematoma caused by the impact of his skull slamming into the wall. He'd hit his head so forcefully, the blow caused a rupture of the middle meningeal artery supplying the brain.

His cranial cavity was flooded with blood. The mass expanded, occupying the small space between the brain's meningeal coverings and the bony braincase. This caused the pressure exerted on the brain to rise precipitously, as the immovable skull could no longer accommodate the expanding blood mass. The brain was compressed and compromised to the point where its vital functions shut down.

The autopsy report noted no brain tumor or any other physical cause for his psychiatrically decompensated state.

It was one of the strangest suicides in the hospital's history.

As I put the report down on my desk, I recalled one cop having said, *"This guy's off the wall."*

The prescience of that statement was chilling.

John Doe was determined to die.

The wall was the only means by which he could achieve his goal on a locked psychiatric ward, completely restrained in a straitjacket, with an orderly clasping his arm.

Having lost all hope, John Doe found a way to die.

And we had failed to save him from himself.

Afterword

John Doe's death brings to mind certain medicolegal issues relating to a hospital's obligations toward a patient, whether on a medical, surgical, or psychiatric ward.

Though it doesn't occur with great frequency, severely ill patients occasionally manage to kill themselves while on strictly supervised, locked psychiatric wards. I've encountered situations where patients, using a sheet, or an article of clothing, have hung themselves in a shower stall. Others have jimmied open a locked Plexiglas window and jumped to their deaths or sustained severe injuries in their attempts to die.

People intent on killing themselves can find a way to do so, despite a hospital's best efforts at preventing suicide.

These cases invariably come to court as civil lawsuits brought by the deceased patient's family or estate against the hospital. The suit alleges the hospital's negligence caused the patient's death.

A brief explanation of the legal principles involved will shed light on the obligations hospitals have toward their patients.

Under the law, when a hospital admits a person to one of its wards, it assumes certain irrefutable responsibilities.

A very important legal doctrine is known as *in loco parentis*. This Latin phrase means *in the place of the parent*.

Under this principle, the responsible party, whether an individual or institution, temporarily assumes parental rights, duties, and obligations toward someone under its care. It applies to places like hospitals, schools, day care facilities, and summer camps, requiring these entities to provide a safe and protective environment for their charges.

This doctrine mandates that hospitals shelter and protect their patients.

When you enter a general hospital, you are bedridden; you cannot control who enters your room or with whom you share the space; you may be heavily medicated, or perhaps you're even lying in bed unconscious. You might be given the wrong medication, resulting in a harmful or even lethal reaction to it. In a very real way, you're completely exposed to the carelessness of others, and you have few defenses.

When you enter a psychiatric ward, you're rendered even more vulnerable by the situation itself. You're living on a ward with disturbed people, some of whom can act in aggressive or dangerous ways. Your own mental illness, by its very nature, renders you vulnerable to acting on destructive impulses, whether directed toward yourself or others. Here, too, if you're given the wrong medication the result could be catastrophic. Again, as on a medical or surgical ward, you're exquisitely vulnerable to the actions or irresponsible inaction of others.

The hospital, like a school, must protect those under its care, just as a parent must safeguard a child.

In a very real way, John Doe's situation mandated that the hospital assume parental obligations while he was on the ward.

The second legal doctrine applicable in John Doe's case is *respondeat superior*, which is Latin for *let the master answer.*

This common-law doctrine makes an employer (the principal) liable for the actions of an employee (the agent), when the actions take place within the scope of the employee's work situation. The legal theory behind *respondeat superior* is the employer controls the employee's behaviors and must assume responsibility for his or her actions.

In keeping with *respondeat superior*, Mr. Johnson was acting as the hospital's agent while working within the scope of his employment. Ultimately, the hospital was responsible for Mr. Johnson's act, which may have involved an omission of some kind, or another form of negligence. Mr. Johnson may not have been strong enough to restrain John Doe. Should this have been recognized by the staff (myself included)? Should we have assigned two younger, stronger aides to accompany him down the hallway? Would two muscular men have been sufficient manpower to prevent this tragedy from occurring?

These questions are, in essence, answered by the legal rule of evidence known as *res ipsa loquitor*, which is Latin for *the thing speaks for itself.*

This rule infers that the defendant—the hospital—was negligent, because the cause of the patient's death was in the defendant's exclusive control and would not have occurred without some form of negligence on the part of the hospital. Other examples of *res ipsa loquitor* are a surgeon leaving a sponge inside a patient's abdomen during surgery; a heavy object falling from a building's window, injuring someone on the sidewalk; or two

trains speeding toward each other on the same track and collid-
ing. In all these situations, the very fact that the incident occurred
is, in and of itself, an indication of negligence on the part of the
person or people in charge.

Given the legal principles involved, no matter how well inten-
tioned the hospital's employees were, in court the facility would
be found negligent in caring for a patient placed in its custody.

The institution failed in its obligation to provide a safe haven
for John Doe.

Surprisingly, no one ever brought suit against the hospital in
this case.

The Family and Me

While working as an attending psychiatrist on the wards, I was given a hospital-based office for treating my own patients when my work shift was over. Though hospitalized patients had compelling stories to tell, my private practice also provided a startling view of the unexpected.

One day I received a call from a former classmate. Vincent and I had met on the first day of medical school, standing over a cadaver in the gross anatomy lab. We became good friends, as do many physicians who together experienced the fascinating exploration of a human body.

Vinzy became an internist, and we referred patients to each other, building our respective practices.

"Joey's an interesting guy," Vinzy said. "Maybe you can help him with some family problems."

A week later Joey P. entered my office. He was a thirty-two-year-old man, dressed casually in gray slacks, a burgundy turtleneck, and black loafers. He had a fleshy face, dark eyes, brown, neatly barbered hair with long sideburns, and a trim mustache—which was very much the style in those days. He sported rings on three fingers and a gold chain around his neck. He lived in Queens and had an Italian surname. A smile formed on his lips as he sat in the chair facing mine.

"Maybe Vinny was right," he said. "You look like the kind of guy I can talk to."

"What brings you here?" I asked.

"Well, I got problems with my father. He's a tough son of a bitch, and it isn't easy workin' for him."

I nodded, knowing from firsthand experience how a family business could brim with discord. I'd learned that lesson when, before medical school, I worked briefly for an uncle who was partnered up with a cousin. It was tooth and nail all day every day. And some patients told similar stories about their family ventures. Being in business with relatives could be a recipe for disaster.

"Tell me about it."

"My father's a real ballbuster," Joey continued. "He's on top of me all the time, never lets up. And he doesn't give me the authority to carry out my responsibilities."

"What kind of business is it?"

"We're in the construction business," he said, shifting in his chair.

"Tell me more."

"He jumps all over me about handling subcontractors even though I know exactly what to do. He goes over every detail again and again. Repeats himself endlessly. Then, if the job doesn't go the way he wants, he yells at me in front of everyone."

It sounded like many family businesses: the tension-filled, father-son dynamic seeped into everything. It bred friction, arguments, and simmering resentment—all inimical to any commercial venture—and wreaked havoc on relationships.

"Like last week," Joey went on, "he told me to get in touch with this guy about a job. He gave me all the details—hook, line, and sinker. So I tell this guy everything. I dot the i's and cross the t's. And what happens? The guy screws up—big-time. So it's my fault? I get yelled at. Everybody sees me gettin' chewed out, like a kid.

"I gotta tell ya, Doc, I feel like I'm ten years old when I'm with him. I end up lookin' like a lackey. And now? Nobody listens to me anymore. They wanna hear everythin' from my father."

Joey described an assortment of degrading incidents where his father had—in not-so-subtle ways—emasculated him in front of employees. We spent an hour talking, during which I got plenty of history about Joey, his mother, and his father.

Joey was an only child. His mother doted on him, in contrast to his father—a rough-hewn man who'd been born "on the other side." From Joey's description, his father was volatile, impatient, and intolerant. He could fly into combustible rages at the slightest departure from his instructions.

"He's always on my case, no matter what I do."

"It's tough to be a son *and* a partner," I said.

"I'm thinkin' of gettin' outta the business."

"And do what?"

"I dunno. I'm stuck. I guess that's why I'm here. Maybe you can help me get away from him, so I can . . . I'd like to be my own man."

In some ways Joey emulated his father: he talked in a gritty patois derived from the mean streets of his neighborhood. Sitting face-to-face and talking with Joey reminded me of my own rough-and-tumble upbringing. Joey was a likable guy with a ready laugh. He radiated warmth, was verbal and intelligent, had a sense of humor, and seemed motivated to deal with his problems. He might benefit from a few months of counseling— from sessions designed to help him see a bit deeper into what was really going on.

He needed to explore and understand more about his dependency on his parents. We agreed to meet once weekly.

Over the next few weeks Joey came regularly to the sessions. It was obvious he was comfortable talking with me, and other elements of his life emerged.

"I'm not a kid, anymore . . . and I'm really thinkin' of movin' out," he said.

"That's not a bad idea."

"My mother wants me to get married. She says it'll help me grow up."

"What does she mean by that?"

"Ah, you know . . . she doesn't wanna do my laundry anymore. She thinks I'm spoiled."

"Are you?"

"Yeah, maybe so," he said with a quick laugh. "I got a good thing at home. Nobody's gonna cook like my mother; and ya know what, Doc? I'll never have it as good as I do at home. But my father . . . that's another story."

"Have you ever worked for anyone else?"

"Nah, I began with him right outta high school."

It struck me that despite Joey's talk about "getting away" from his father's clutches, his lack of experience outside the family business left him with few viable options. He seemed stuck in time and place—emotionally and occupationally.

Over the next two months, the focus of the sessions became clear: Joey was the "golden boy" who would never leave the security and comfort of his childhood home.

"I guess I got mixed feelings about movin' out," he admitted. "I got everything I could ever want there, so why look for somethin' else?"

"Because the price you end up paying is feeling you get no respect."

"You mean like Rodney Dangerfield?" he said with a chortle.

"He makes a living by joking about it. But you . . . Though you have a good thing at home, you resent being made to feel like a kid."

He squinted and nodded. "You know, I was thinkin' . . . even my name, Joey . . . That's what everyone calls me. It's never Joe or Joseph. It's always *Joey*. It's a kid's name."

He was getting the message.

"Actually, Doc, I shoulda been more up front with you."

"Up front about what?" I asked, perplexed by his statement.

"About my father and the family . . . the business." He sighed and looked at me, as though waiting for encouragement to say more.

I remained silent.

"We're into more than just construction," he said. "We also have some interest in a garbage hauling company and . . . a few other concerns."

"What other concerns?"

"I can't really say right now."

Not being naive, I had a good idea what Joey was trying to tell me.

"Actually, some of it's a little on the shady side," he added. "I can't get into specifics, but I'm sure you know what I mean."

Though he never said it outright, it was abundantly clear: Joey's father held some sort of position—perhaps he was an underboss—in a New York City crime family. I tried not to jump to conclusions, but felt certain Joey's father had ties to the New York underworld.

And equally clear was the real possibility Joey—working for his father—was in some way "connected" to the New York mob scene as well.

Was I treating the son of a mobster?

If my conjecture was correct, what would happen if certain ugly realities emerged during our sessions—facts or inferences about which I would never willingly inquire?

Would I then become part of a conspiracy of silence?

I consoled myself with a simple notion: Joey's treatment was time-limited and focused on one major issue—his dependency on his parents. Despite my rationalization, I began to feel uneasy about Joey's probable criminal connections. My sixth sense was signaling to me that this patient could spell trouble.

One evening in mid-July—about three months into the therapy—Joey entered the consultation room. As he sat down, his lips curled into a knowing smile.

I sensed something unusual would emerge—maybe some kernel of newly realized insight, or perhaps he'd finally decided to leave the nest and look for a place of his own.

Usually, Joey began talking the moment he entered the office, even before taking a seat; but this session started differently. He walked to his chair in silence, settled in, and fixed his eyes on me. He leaned forward—still, not a word passed his lips.

I waited, uncertain what to expect.

In a voice barely above a whisper, and one I can still conjure in my mind to this day, he uttered the words:

"You wanna know who clipped Carmine Galante . . . ?"

My heart thrashed in my chest and my skin felt electrified.

Joey was referring to a mob rubout that had occurred only a few days earlier, on July 12, 1979.

It was big news about which newspaper headlines shrieked.

Carmine "Cigar" Galante, an acting boss in the Bonanno crime family, had finished eating lunch on the backyard patio at Joe and Mary's Italian-American Restaurant on Knickerbocker Avenue in Brooklyn. Galante was dining with two Bonanno gang members, along with his Sicilian bodyguards.

Suddenly, three ski-masked men burst into the restaurant and strode brazenly out to the patio. They opened fire with shotguns and handguns, killing three of the men instantly, including Galante.

Everyone in New York City knew about the hit. The story was on television and radio and was plastered all over the newspapers. Front-page photos in the *New York Daily News* and *New York Post* showed Galante—dead as a proverbial doornail—sprawled on the patio pavement. His head was crooked against a low brick wall. Blood was splattered everywhere. One bullet had blown completely through Galante's left eye socket.

The ugliness of the photographs included a bizarre anomaly: protruding from the dead Galante's clenched teeth was a still-smoking stogie.

You wanna know who clipped Carmine Galante?

Joey's question echoed in my head. Though every nerve in my body felt like it was firing, I was completely mute. Frozen.

You wanna know who clipped Carmine Galante?

Thoughts streaked through my mind in a shuttling profusion. I sat there in stunned silence, paralyzed.

It was an offer I could *definitely* refuse.

"No. I don't want to know," I heard myself croak, but was at a loss about what—if anything—else to say.

Joey nodded and then calmly proceeded to talk about his home life as though nothing out of the ordinary had been said.

Thoughts blitzed through my mind so precipitously, I barely heard a word Joey uttered. Visions of mob goons, rubouts, and threats—even images of Brando, Pacino, and Caan from *The Godfather*—streaked through my head. Did Joey's mobster father know his son was seeing a psychiatrist? Did he know Joey was seeing *me*? If so, what on earth did he think Joey was telling me behind closed doors? How much did—or would—I learn about the family business? About payoffs to judges, politicians, city inspectors, about the rackets, extortions, and murders?

Patients tell their shrinks things they would never tell anyone else. After all, everything said is held in the strictest confidence. And to top it off, Joey was an extremely talkative guy—at times even verbose.

A sickening realization hit me: no matter what was—or *wasn't*—said in our private meetings, someone in the "family" might *think* I heard far too much about the family business, that certain secrets had been revealed.

And then what might happen?

To me?

Why hadn't I asked myself these questions earlier, when I had a nascent inkling of what Joey's family business was all about?

Although this occurred long before the fictional Dr. Melfi treated Tony in *The Sopranos*, I was faced with the same potentially disastrous situation.

What was I supposed to do?

My profession demanded I cultivate trust and confidence with Joey, but in speaking with him, I might be privy to a description of a wide assortment of illegalities. I was ethically bound by the doctor-patient relationship to keep his confidence, but did Joey's family know that?

When Joey left the office, I was barely able to recall anything he'd said other than:

"You wanna know who clipped Carmine Galante?"

What could—or should—I do? Had I been party to information implicating my patient in some criminal conspiracy? Had I learned more than I realized about some mob-orchestrated plot to commit murder? If so, what could or should happen? Did I have an obligation to report something to the police? Should I call a lawyer? Or should I simply say nothing—to anyone?

Did confidentiality between my patient and me mean I had an obligation to keep quiet about whatever Joey implied or told me? Exactly what were my ethical obligations in this insane scenario?

Was I in danger?

My hands trembled as I picked up the telephone.

The next day, as arranged, I went to see the man I'd called. He'd been one of my case supervisors during my residency at Manhattan Hospital.

I'd already become interested in forensic psychiatry and viewed Dr. Walter Conway as a mentor. In medical-legal circles, he was something of a legend. His keen mind and depth of knowledge made him a valuable consultant to attorneys in both civil and criminal cases. He'd been called upon in hundreds of situations where psychiatry and the law intersected. On some occasions he'd been consulted by the police who were seeking a psychological profile of a serial killer.

His office had a lobby entrance in a white-glove building on Park Avenue in the Eighties. Dr. Conway's consultation room reminded me of photographs of Freud's Vienna office at 19 Berggasse Street. Sepia-toned photographs, prints, and drawings adorned the mahogany-paneled walls. Glass-encased bookshelves held rows of gilt-edged, leather-bound volumes relating to medicine, psychiatry, and law. A battalion of pre-Columbian statuettes stood on his desk. Elaborate Kashan rugs covered the floor.

Dr. Conway had steel-gray hair and deep blue eyes. He dressed in old tweeds, wore a pocket watch, and smoked a meerschaum pipe.

The room and the man were very Old World, and both were redolent of Cavendish pipe smoke.

We sat facing each other. I explained the situation, telling Conway about the dilemma into which I'd suddenly been thrust. I didn't mention Joey's name or provide any identifying details.

Dr. Conway listened carefully and then leaned back in his leather chair. "This young man wasn't completely honest with you, was he?" he asked. "He didn't mention the mob connection until well into the therapy, correct?"

"Yes. I learned about it a few months later."

"So, he may have thought you wouldn't want to treat him if you'd known of his connections, yes?"

"Very possibly."

"Telling you his father was in the construction business and not mentioning anything else was a lie of omission, wasn't it?"

"Yes."

Dr. Conway nodded. "You did the right thing, telling him you didn't want to know about the murder."

"For selfish reasons, I didn't want to know a thing."

"Call it selfish or call it smart. It was the best thing to do."

I nodded, knowing my instincts had been right. "Am I obligated to inform the authorities?"

"No," replied Conway. "Generally the law makes an exception when it comes to psychiatrists and their patients," Conway said. "There's enormous weight placed on the issue of confidentiality in these circumstances—whether it's the doctor-patient relationship or the priest-penitent situation.

"But let me explain something," he added. "If a patient tells you he *intends* to commit a crime you're obligated to inform the authorities. If you don't, you could be considered an accessory before the fact. In fact, if you reasonably *suspect* a patient will harm someone, you're obligated to inform the intended victim and the authorities. The famous *Tarasoff* decision made that very clear."

"I'm somewhat familiar with the case."

"It was a watershed case in psychiatry," Conway said. "In 1974, Tatiana Tarasoff was a young woman at the University of California. A male student made advances, but she rebuffed him. He became distraught and pursued her—relentlessly. Basically, he was stalking her. A friend urged him to get treatment, so he began seeing a psychologist at the university clinic.

"The psychologist thought this young man was very disturbed, especially when he confided that he wanted to kill Ms. Tarasoff. The psychologist had the campus police arrest the man, and he was confined to the university hospital. But he was discharged, even though he was diagnosed as dangerously psychotic.

"The result?" Conway said with raised eyebrows. "He stabbed Ms. Tarasoff to death. Her parents sued the university, claiming they were negligent in discharging the patient without having warned Ms. Tarasoff about the danger he presented. The

California Supreme Court made it very clear: a mental health professional has a duty not only to a patient but also to anyone threatened by that patient."

"Wasn't that decision appealed?" I asked.

"Yes, but it was upheld by the appellate court," Conway said. "And the decision's been adopted by most states. The majority opinion said, and I quote, 'The protection of the patient-psychotherapist confidential communications must yield to the extent to which disclosure is essential to avert danger to others. The protective privilege ends where public peril begins.'"

Conway sucked on his pipe. His head was shrouded by a blue-gray corona of aromatic smoke.

"But your situation is different," he said. "We're not dealing with a crime *about* to be committed. Your patient claims to have knowledge about a crime that's *already* been committed.

"And you have no idea if he actually knows anything about the murder. He may have been trying to impress you in some adolescent way. After all, emotionally he's still in that stage of development."

Conway paused, tamped his pipe, and leaned back in his chair.

"Basically, you're fine not saying anything. The confidentiality exception holds for you and for this patient. What was said was spoken in confidence, may have no factual basis, and no crime is about to be committed. The *Tarasoff* ruling doesn't apply."

"I don't know if I can go on treating him," I said.

"Understood," Conway said. "That's the next important question. What's your ethical responsibility to him?"

"Do I have an obligation to continue treating him?"

"In the law, the obligation you have toward a patient is called a duty. So, you have a *duty* to a patient, yes?"

"Yes . . ."

"It's a duty to be thorough, to care about the patient's well-being, and to use the most current knowledge available. Your duty includes maintaining a confidential relationship with the patient and not abandoning him."

"Would I be abandoning this patient if I terminate his treatment?"

Conway set his pipe in an ashtray.

"Abandoning the patient? Let me say this: your duty to *this* patient doesn't include *endangering your own life*, which is obviously your concern, yes?"

"Absolutely."

"Then you're under no obligation to continue treating this man."

At the beginning of our next session, trepidation gnawed at me.

"We have to talk very frankly," I began.

He peered at me expectantly.

My heart pounded erratically.

"I can't treat you anymore."

His eyes widened. "Why not, Doc?"

"Because of what you mentioned last session about Galante."

"I really didn't tell you anything."

I felt like I was walking on shards of glass—barefoot.

"You told me enough." My throat closed.

"Enough for what?"

"Enough to make me worry about what your father and his associates might think you tell me in these sessions. I could be in danger."

"But what we say in here is private. It's just between you and me."

"But other people know you come here, right?"

"Only one or two."

"We don't know what they *think* you tell me."

Joey closed his eyes and nodded. He got the point.

There was an uncomfortable silence. It went on for what seemed a very long time. Finally, he said, "Hey, Doc. I like you. I don't wanna see nothin' happen to you."

"That's why we can't meet anymore."

Joey's eyes met mine, and he smiled.

A feeling of relief swept through me.

That was the last session we had.

Afterword

I've thought about Joey ever since my relatively brief interface with him—not only because I perceived a possible threat to my well-being but because of another important reason.

I became aware of something that's stayed with me throughout the years: when you take someone on in treatment—no matter how time-limited or focused the sessions may be—in a very tangible way, you enter into and become part of that person's life. Yes, you avoid becoming part of the patient's "real" life—you don't have any contact outside the office—but even if only in fantasy, the person perceives you as playing a crucial role in his or her affairs. The therapist-patient relationship is a very special and intimate one.

I also learned something else from my contact with Joey.

As a therapist, you ultimately have very little control over the treatment outcome. There are many variables—known and unknown—affecting how well or how poorly a patient does by virtue of counseling. You must be satisfied knowing you did the best you could under whatever unpredictable circumstances may have prevailed at the time of treatment.

I hoped that over the brief period of time we worked together Joey managed to develop enough insight to make some meaningful changes in his home life.

As far as Joey's *work* was concerned, my hopes were unlike those I'd ever had with any patient.

Behind Bars

After completing my residency, I was hired as an attending psychiatrist at the hospital, where my responsibilities involved working on the wards and supervising psychiatric residents, psychology interns, and social workers. As a newly minted psychiatrist, I enjoyed much of the work, but the most intriguing and challenging venue was the prison ward where I sometimes examined patients.

Every form of madness was housed behind the floor-to-ceiling bars confronting you as you stepped off the dedicated elevator serving only the prison ward. A New York City corrections officer was posted at the entrance and controlled access to the area.

Many of the inmates, psychotic to an extreme degree, included agitated, impulse-driven criminals; pumped-up, hyperverbal drug addicts; shameless psychopathic killers; inveterate food-throwers and feces-flingers; remorseless child-killers; wife-beaters; robbers and rapists—even a man who'd killed his six-year-old daughter, believing she was the devil in disguise.

Doctors, nurses, or the police were the only ones allowed beyond the outer bars located fifteen feet from the elevator door. The unmistakable funk of excrement and unwashed bodies assaulted your nostrils as you passed beyond the prison bars. Shrieks, threats, and curses filled the air. The ward's atmosphere was one of madness welded to menace.

The majority of prisoners were sent from the Rikers Island Correctional Facility—a pretrial holding complex—after exhibiting bizarre behavior while incarcerated. Some were being evaluated for competency to stand trial. Others were remanded for examination regarding an insanity defense.

I'd been an attending psychiatrist for a number of years when I received a telephone call from Dr. Donald Wilson, the hospital's chief of forensic services. He was a crusty, no-nonsense man who'd long ago made the prison ward his home turf. "I'd like to refer a case to you," he said. "Ordinarily, I'd do the evaluation, but I don't have time. It will involve traveling to the Fishkill Correctional Facility in Beacon, New York, to examine a prisoner. Are you interested?"

"Could be. Tell me more."

"It's unusual because the inmate's filed a civil suit against the state. I was contacted by the defense counsel for New York State."

"Is he suing for prosecutorial misconduct?"

"No. His guilt was never in doubt. He's doing twenty-five to life for armed robbery. He's been in maximum security for three years now. He claims there're particulates—mold or dust, whatever—in the prison air ducts that've caused him to develop breathing problems."

"And he's suing the state?"

"Yes. Even as a prisoner he has the constitutional right to his day in court, and he's suing for damages to his lungs."

"Why're they asking for a psychiatric evaluation?"

"Two reasons. First, the judge wants to know if he's capable of representing himself. He's filed the suit on a *pro se* basis—acting as his own attorney. And second, the defendant—in this case, New York State—wants to know if he's delusional, if he has some psychotic idea about poisons being in the prison air. If that's it, the state will make a motion for summary judgment."

"Sounds like it could be interesting."

"Yes, and the state will pay your fee for reviewing records, traveling to Beacon, examining the guy, and preparing a report for exchange with the plaintiff, namely, the inmate himself. It means taking most of a day out of your schedule. If you're willing to do it, I'll contact the state's attorneys and make sure they send you his records and legal filings."

Two weeks later I drove to Beacon, New York.

On the way I felt a sense of anticipation about interviewing plaintiff-prisoner Aaron J.

Based on the intricacy of his handwritten legal filings, it was clear Aaron J. had spent countless hours in the prison library, soaking up volumes from scholarly articles and books. His legal papers—including his bill of particulars, a detailed complaint alleging the state's negligence and his damages—were jotted with a number two graphite pencil and organized in neat, block print. The documents conveyed in precise, lawyerly verbiage his allegations about the prison's duct system and its allegedly contaminated air. He claimed it had caused severe respiratory problems that continued to plague him and would do so into the future.

He'd obviously used his prison time to become the proverbial jailhouse lawyer.

But was he insane, like so many other prisoners I'd evaluated on the prison ward? Was he a litigiously paranoid individual?

If so, that could change the complexion of the case. And if he *was* psychotic, where precisely did he fit in the spectrum of mental illnesses? Did he perceive the world through a distorted paranoid lens, rendering the most innocuous surroundings—the very air he breathed—potentially lethal?

Did he believe some nefarious plot was afoot to poison or incapacitate him?

Did he believe the state was persecuting him for unimaginably evil reasons? Such delusional thinking wasn't unusual on the prison ward, and it could certainly happen at Fishkill.

Despite the logical and orderly presentation of his bill of particulars, would Aaron J.'s words be little more than garbled word salad—a jumbled outpouring of indecipherable ramblings? Would he perseverate on the avalanche of injustices allegedly done to him by the police, the lawyers, the malevolent machinery of the state's prison system, and the entire world?

Did he hear voices? See visions? Was he a prophet? An apostle? Was he the reincarnation of Moses, or Jesus, or could he be—in his own perverse reality—the living embodiment of God?

Or was he a convicted felon with worsening breathing problems who was rationally pursuing legal action against the state?

With these conceivable scenarios in mind, I drove north toward the Hudson River town of Beacon.

As the highway descended to the river at Newburgh, the Fishkill Correctional Facility came into view.

The prison grounds looked like something out of a Hieronymus Bosch painting. Constructed in 1896, the complex had an eerily nightmarish appearance.

A series of low-lying redbrick buildings sat on a vast, treeless expanse surrounded by rows of chain-link fences stretching to the horizon. The enclosures were topped by gleaming coils of concertina wire. Additional rolls of razor wire—helical battalions of sharp-edged steel—surrounded the perimeter of the outermost fence.

Against a gloomy sky, the buildings with their conical roofs topping round guard-tower turrets, combined with the formidable walls and fences, underscored the prison's fortress-like impenetrability.

The guards at the main entrance had been told to expect me.

Despite this advance notice and my being there at the behest of the state, I was subjected to a mandatory search. I'd thought it would be a perfunctory frisk, but I was wrong.

My identification was checked, as were the contents of my wallet and the court papers allowing admittance to the prison. I was asked a series of questions, designed, I imagined, to ensure I wasn't an imposter. I was wanded and then I walked through a metal detector and was patted down; my pockets were searched; and I was told to remove my shoes and belt, which were examined. My briefcase was opened and thoroughly checked.

A burly guard escorted me along a seemingly endless, windowless corridor. The walls were cinder block and smelled of mold; the ceiling and floor were poured concrete. As we neared an electronically controlled gate, a buzzer sounded and the gate slid open and then closed behind us. We passed through the second set of mobile floor-to-ceiling doors.

"What a place," I said to the guard.

"It's like being in hell," he replied, shaking his head.

We walked along what seemed another interminable corridor—so stark and forbidding, our voices echoed as we talked.

"I'm trying to imagine what it's like spending years here," I said.

"I work here five days a week and it gets to me."

"At least you leave at the end of your shift."

"You got it. These guys . . . they go nowhere."

"This place could drive you crazy if you were sane when you first got here," I said.

The guard nodded.

Another electronic door opened and then shut behind us. We were being swallowed up—walking deeper into the belly of the beast. The gray cinder-block walls, cement floors, lack of windows, and sickly fluorescent lighting made for a sense of dislocation. The corridor seemed to grow colder as we walked.

We passed an interior courtyard. A group of newly arrived prisoners, chained to each other, was being led from a prison van. Still wearing civilian clothes, they were lined up, about to be inspected for contraband. That would, no doubt, include a body-cavity search, meaning they would be forced to strip naked and squat, while a guard—using a mirror on a pole—would inspect their rectums. They would then be issued prison garb.

The guard escorted me through another series of impregnable-looking doors; we climbed a short stairway and then arrived at the medical unit. I was introduced to an administrator, who said the examination would take place in a locked room down the hall.

If I were claustrophobic, the experience would have been intolerable. As it was, I was itching to bolt from this enclosed world of bars, buzzers, corridors, guards, and sliding doors.

Nothing could have prepared me for the horrific atmosphere of prison. Despite having looked forward to this experience on my drive to Fishkill, I now wanted nothing more than to burst through the outer doors and escape.

But that wasn't to be—at least not for the next few hours. I'd be locked in a suffocating cubicle with a possibly psychotic inmate who was suing the State of New York.

And by extension, I represented the very entity he was suing.

The administrator handed me a device. "Attach this to your belt," he instructed. "It's a body alarm. If you think trouble's brewing, just press the red button and an alarm will sound. You'll also be in radio contact with the guards. They'll come immediately."

What did I get myself into?

A chill came over me. "Is this guy violent?"

"He hasn't been, but you never know. Let me warn you," the administrator added. "*Any* felon in this institution is capable of violence. These guys aren't your buddies, no matter how friendly they may seem. They can't be trusted. Ever. You could be shanked in the blink of an eye."

"What about Aaron J.?"

"He's been thoroughly searched. He's clean. But stay vigilant."

I definitely regretted my willingness to do this evaluation.

I had no idea what to expect.

Would Aaron J. be some tattoo-covered, pumped-up, muscle-bound guy able to bench-press twice his body weight? Would he be consumed by barely controlled hatred—especially for those he perceived as representatives of the state's power? Would I become the target of the loathing he no doubt harbored toward those who'd imprisoned him? Would he be aggressive? Would he relate to me with contempt? He was serving twenty-five to life for an armed robbery during which a cop had been shot. How potentially violent—or insane—would this guy be?

I sat in a chair at a small table in a bare, windowless, locked room. Brightly lit by recessed fluorescent tubes, the enclosure seemed sterile, devoid of life. I wondered why they'd locked the door while I sat there alone.

I waited, feeling my pulse throb in my wrists.

The sound of a key in the door's locking mechanism caught my attention.

The door opened.

Aaron J. was escorted into the room by a guard. The officer slipped out of the room and locked the door.

I rose to greet the prisoner.

Aaron J. was a slight, wiry, thirty-year-old black man. A soul patch perched beneath his lower lip. His face was thin; his eyes were bright with anticipation. He wore an orange jumpsuit, no hand-cuffs or shackles. To my relief, he smiled as we shook hands. His handshake was warm and firm; it seemed genuine, and he looked pleasant enough. He was nothing like I'd imagined he might be. Still, after the administrator's warning, every nerve ending in my body was firing in a skin-tingling frenzy.

"So, Doc, you're gonna see if I'm crazy?" he said with a quick grin.

I smiled weakly and beckoned him to sit across from me at the table.

He settled into the chair, leaned back, clasped his hands behind his head, and stared at me. He was studying me. Did he perceive me as an adversary, someone who would try to deep-six his case? Was he sizing me up, just as many attorneys in courtrooms had done in the past?

I was reminded he was not only an inmate but also a plaintiff and was acting as his own lawyer, if I determined he was competent enough to do so. Anything I said or asked could be used during his cross-examination of me in open court.

I was in the strange position of being both the examiner and the examinee.

"So where do we begin?" he asked.

His tone was neutral, bordering on friendly. I felt the tension dissipating. Slightly.

"Do you know why we're meeting today?" I asked.

Though I'd been told he was completely aware of the purpose of our meeting, I had to ensure that was true.

"Of course I do, Doc."

"Tell me why."

"The state wants to see if I'm insane, and the judge wants to make sure I can represent myself in court, that's why."

"You're right," I said, knowing the interview would be done with the inmate's informed consent. "You also know I've been asked to prepare a report that'll be entered into the court proceedings, right?"

"That's correct. And I'll get a copy of it."

"Right," I said, well aware Aaron J. knew the ins and outs of CPLR, Civil Practice Law and Rules. "I've read your legal papers. They're very well done and explain your lawsuit completely. So the judge's worry about self-representation doesn't seem to be a concern." My voice was surprisingly steady—not quavering.

"Thank you," he replied with a sigh. "I've had plenty of time to learn the legal trade."

I nodded, thinking of the unending stretch of time Aaron J. would face in this hellish place known as Fishkill.

"Why don't you tell me about your breathing problems?"

In a relaxed manner, he described his difficulties since being incarcerated at Fishkill.

"After I'd been here a few months, I noticed I woke up every morning with phlegm and mucous in my throat. And recently I've been short of breath. It's worse in the mornings and evenings," he said and then coughed into his closed fist. "Excuse me," he added. The social propriety seemed to relieve my tension even more.

"It's gotten so bad, I have rib pain from coughing all the time." He continued, detailing his physical difficulties. There was nothing odd or bizarre about his description of the problem. He didn't attribute it to some malevolent intention by prison personnel or other inmates. It was a realistic description of his physical difficulties. It sounded very much like seasonal or other allergies. Or maybe he'd developed chronic bronchitis. After all, the medical records said he was a smoker, sucking in a pack of cigarettes each day for years.

But his physical condition would be evaluated by a pulmonologist; my task was different.

As I listened to him recount his troubles, certain things seemed clear: he wasn't hallucinating and harbored no evidence of delusional thinking. He was neither grandiose nor suspicious. There was nothing ostensibly psychotic about Aaron J.; nor was there anything remotely sinister about the man. Had we not been thrown together under extraordinary circumstances and locked inside a prison's maximum-security block, he'd seem like an ordinary guy describing his troubles.

But sometimes you must dig deeper to excavate a patient's mental pathology.

After he described his breathing problems, Aaron J. talked a bit about his life at Fishkill. It was constricting, confining, even suffocating, except for his excursions to the prison library, where he spent every free hour possible, reading the law—civil and criminal. He talked a bit about his reading. It was clear he was an intuitive and very intelligent man.

"Tell me a little about yourself, about your life before this place."

He smiled and shrugged. "What can I tell ya, Doc? I never knew my parents. I never had anyone who really cared. I'm not making excuses for myself, but it was tough going."

"How so?"

He clasped his hands together on the table. "Me and my sister were separated when I was three. We got farmed out to a bunch of foster homes. I spent the first twelve years of my life in six different homes. Some were okay, but a few of 'em, well . . . I don't wanna go into it. Let's just say I learned from an early age that the world isn't a great place. Some people are just born into rotten circumstances. Ya know what I mean?"

I nodded, knowing there was very likely abuse and neglect in the foster homes.

"There was one guy in particular . . . If I ran into him today, I'd . . . well, we won't talk about it, okay?"

His lips tightened; his cheeks bunched as his teeth clenched, and he looked down at the table.

I kept silent.

He looked up at me and inhaled deeply. "I learned that life on the streets was easier than in those foster homes. I did what a lot of the brothers do; I fell in with the wrong crowd. You know how it is for a kid. I learned to value all the wrong things. I looked up to the wrong kinda people. At first it was playing hooky, tossin' dice, smoking dope, and some petty stuff—you know, stealing from stores, crap like that."

He shook his head and sighed.

"And one thing led to another. So, before I knew it, I ended up on Rikers, and from there I was sent upstate and did two years for burglary. When I got out, things weren't any better. I got only myself to blame, Doc. I made bad choices, especially when I joined up with two guys who were into armed robberies."

He paused. For a moment a distant look formed in his eyes.

"So, we held up a convenience store," he said, "and before I knew what was goin' down, the cops show up and shots get fired. I didn't have a piece, but that don't matter. I was in on it. One cop was wounded, and the clerk nearly died from a gunshot to the stomach."

He shook his head.

"So here I am, doin' twenty-five to life."

His story seemed pathetic, predictable, and troubling. But aside from its content, I was tasked with evaluating his form of speech and thinking. After all, this was a diagnostic psychiatric examination, a medicolegal excursion in the context of his litigation agenda.

Aaron J. spoke in a logical, goal-directed, and coherent way. There was no loosening of associations; each word flowed rationally from that preceding it and segued seamlessly into those following. He was verbal without being voluble. There was no evidence of disordered thinking. His vocabulary was quite sophisticated for a man who'd never gone beyond the second year of high school. His insight about himself was good, and his judgment was sound: he could capably predict the outcome of any action he might take. He was obviously intelligent. There were no cognitive problems: his memory and thinking processes were completely intact.

Everything he said made sense. I was compelled by his story and didn't feel he was playing me or taking me for a ride. There was something genuine about him.

It was a wasted life.

We discussed his lawsuit and the issues he wanted addressed by the court.

"Hey, Doc, I know all about presenting a case to a jury," he said, and then recited every step in a trial, from the attorneys' opening statements to closing arguments. He discussed civil procedure and the rules of evidence a jury could use to reach its verdict in a civil case. "And I know I'll only have to show the state's liability and my damages by a *preponderance* of evidence, not beyond a reasonable doubt, like in a criminal trial," he added. "The bar's set much lower in a civil proceeding."

His knowledge of the legal process was impressive. He'd done his due diligence.

As he went on, Aaron J. sounded like a seasoned personal injury attorney. There was no doubt he could competently comport himself in a court of law.

After we'd talked for more than an hour, I said, "Aaron, you've really learned a lot about the law and how to apply it. It's quite an accomplishment."

He smiled broadly, obviously appreciating my comment.

"You're a very smart guy," I added.

"Hey, even if ya think I'm crazy, that doesn't mean I'm stupid, right?"

Nodding, I smiled.

"Hey, Doc, wanna hear a joke?"

"Sure," I answered, not knowing what to expect.

"You hear the one about a guy who gets a flat tire in front of an insane asylum?"

I shook my head and leaned back in the chair. It was so strange: I was in a locked room with a maximum-security-prison inmate, about to hear a joke about a guy in an insane asylum.

Aaron J. began. "The driver gets out of his car, sees he's got a flat, and changes the tire. But when he puts on the spare, he can't find the four lug nuts from the tire he took off. He doesn't know what to do.

"A guy calls to him from a window of the insane asylum. 'Hey,' yells the guy. 'Slip the spare tire on. Then take one lug nut off each of the other three tires, put 'em on the spare, and drive to a repair shop; pick up four more lug nuts and put one on each tire.'

"'That's a smart idea,' the guy calls back.

"The nut yells back, 'Hey, I might be crazy, but *I'm not stupid like you!*'"

We both laughed heartily as he slapped his palm on the table. I knew I'd be repeating the joke to hospital colleagues.

I really liked him. Our back-and-forth was friendly and easy-going. Never for a moment had I felt the least bit intimidated. Though he knew I'd prepare a report about his state of mind and his competency to represent himself in court—a report that, for all he knew, could run counter to his litigation agenda—I felt he enjoyed our talk, too.

After an hour and a half, it was abundantly clear: Aaron J. was perfectly sane. In fact, I concluded he'd be a formidable adversary in a courtroom. I could imagine him peppering state officials—to whom he'd already issued subpoenas—with a blistering barrage of well-researched and very loaded questions.

I'd completely forgotten we were in a room deep inside the bowels of an impregnable prison's maximum-security block. It struck me like a sledgehammer: I'd had negative expectations of my encounter with Aaron J.—all based on prior experiences with prison inmates at Manhattan Hospital.

Finally, I said, "Lemme ask you something, Aaron. What do you expect to gain by your lawsuit?"

He crossed his arms in front of him; his brow furrowed. "I guess I just wanna make this a better place. After all, Doc, I'm gonna be here a long time. I gotta have something to live for."

"And you hope to do what, prevail in court?"

"I don't know if that'll happen. I know the cards're stacked against me. It'll probably be a kangaroo court. But I'll tell ya this: I don't sit around all day and rot, like most of these guys do. Studying law gives me purpose. I have a reason to put my feet on the floor every morning."

"Looking forward to something's a good thing," I said.

"Every day when I wake up, I can't wait to get to the library. I wanna learn more and more."

"So, you're living to learn . . . to gain knowledge. Maybe even to change a few things around here . . . ?"

He nodded. "That about sums it up, Doc. And maybe, some-day, when I get outta here, I can be a paralegal. That's what I hope to do . . . maybe."

"That's a good thing," I said. "To have hope."

We sat silently for a few moments.

Finally, he said, "So tell me, Doc, am I crazy?"

"You know I can't divulge my findings to a litigant," I said, try-ing to stifle a smile.

"Hey, I'm a litigant, not just an inmate now, right?" he said with a broad grin.

"That's right."

"It's good to have a different label," he said, canting his head. "So, am I a *crazy* litigant?"

"Yeah, crazy like a fox."

"I'm just testin' ya, Doc."

"Did I pass the test?"

"Yeah, Doc. You're a good guy. I like you."

"I like you, too," I said in all earnestness.

He leaned back and laughed. "That's good to hear, Doc." He

slapped his palm on the table once again. "And don't you worry; when this case goes to trial, I'll go easy on ya on cross-examination."

We laughed as I gathered my papers. We both stood. I leaned across the table and we shook hands.

"I'm glad ya came to see me, Doc."

"I'm glad, too. It was a pleasure to meet you."

I walked over to the door and knocked on it.

A moment later the locking mechanism unlatched and the guard appeared.

Aaron J. was ready to be led away.

"Good luck with your litigation," I said.

"Take care, Doc. See ya in court."

As I headed back toward the main entrance, the warm feelings of the time spent with Aaron J. faded and were replaced by the hellish reality of this prison, the place he had to call home.

As I approached my car in the visitors' parking lot, a slight breeze kicked up from the west. The steel-wool-gray clouds had dissipated and the sun shone. I inhaled deeply, relishing the pine-scented fresh air and the freedom of my life.

I never saw Aaron J. again.

The case never came to trial. It probably settled.

Afterword

I've thought about Aaron J. many times since that day we met. Certain things about him and the evaluation have stayed with me all these years.

Recalling I'd expected Aaron J. to be a "typical" inmate in a maximum-security facility, I realized I'd prejudged him—wrongly.

Prejudice is an interesting word—one, I think, not fully considered by most of us.

Literally, the word means to *prejudge* someone or something. It means holding or forming an opinion—either favorable or unfavorable—beforehand, without knowledge, thought, or reason. Expanding the definition a bit, it connotes unreasonable feelings, opinions, or attitudes, especially hostile ones, regarding a person, or an ethnic, a social, or a religious group.

As I look back, there's no doubt I'd prejudged Aaron J. I expected a venomous, even paranoid, individual—seething and ranting with uncontrolled rancor. My expectations were very likely fostered by my exposure to prisoner-patients at Manhattan Hospital and by Aaron J.'s status as a convicted felon.

Yes, I'd been prejudicial in my thinking.

After I spent time with the man—when, by dint of some slight familiarity—he became more than simply a prison inmate to me.

I saw him as a man.

Aaron J. demonstrated remarkable resiliency and adaptive capacity while in prison. With a more auspicious upbringing, he could have become an attorney or a professional in virtually any field. But circumstances beyond his control—coupled with poor choices—created a far different outcome.

I couldn't help but wonder what might have become of me had I been born into Aaron J.'s situation. And I pondered if I'd have been able to adjust to prison and maintain my sanity as well as he had, had our roles and lives been reversed.

Somehow, this pensive, intelligent man was able to maintain purpose and *hope* behind bars.

A Short Memory

When he walked into my office, Ralph virtually filled the doorway. Though he stood about five ten, he weighed a solid two hundred sixty pounds. He'd probably put on twenty pounds of flab over his forty-five years, but was built like the proverbial Mack Truck—mostly solid muscle. He had club-sized hands, and his thick fingers looked like pork sausages. His face was huge and fleshy and had something of a bulldog look. His thinning hair was styled in a partial comb-over.

He wore a tweed sports jacket, black slacks, and a white shirt open at the collar. From the drape of the jacket and the bulge beneath, I surmised he was carrying a pistol. Sure enough, after he lumbered toward the chair and lowered himself to sit across from me, I spied the handle of a holstered revolver protruding from beneath his left armpit.

He must have seen my eyes fix on the weapon. "Don't worry, Doc," he said. "Like I told ya on the phone, I'm a PI, and I'm licensed to carry." He patted the holstered weapon and then shifted his bulk in the chair.

"You said you were having a problem with a relationship," I began.

"Yeah, Doc. It's drivin' me crazy, and I really need some help."

Ralph's having mentioned a problematic relationship indicated a certain level of psychological mindedness. He was sufficiently in touch with his inner emotional life to know he needed help sorting out certain difficulties in relation to another person.

"Tell me about it," I said.

Ralph leaned forward; his elbows rested on his knees. He wrung his hands as he began talking. "Well, it started about six months ago. But lemme back up a little. I been divorced about three years now, and I have an apartment on East Thirty-Ninth Street. I been lonely, but hey, that goes with the territory, right, Doc?"

I nodded, knowing single life in Manhattan—despite the crowds, clubs, bars, and glitter—could be a lonely, isolating existence.

"Anyway, I got a good business goin' with the PI thing. I got lotsa clients and plenty of connections with the NYPD, so I get tons of referrals. The money isn't bad and the cases are like buses: there's always another comin' along." He chortled. "Since I'm runnin' a solo operation, I don't have much time for socializing, if ya know what I mean. I do mostly divorce work. Followin' cheatin' husbands and wives," he said with another quick laugh. "It keeps me busy at nights, goin' to bars and hotels, taking photos of people doin' what they shouldn't be doin'."

"I get the picture," I said with a quick smile.

"You get the picture? Ha, that's a good one, Doc." He laughed and slapped the chair's armrest with a meaty hand. "Yeah, if it wasn't for my camera, I'd be outta business. Anyway, when it first began, I thought it was the biggest stroke of luck ever in my whole life."

"When what first began?"

"Ya see, I met this woman. Laurel's her name. She's a real traffic stopper. Tall, a great body, sexy as hell, and really knows how to please a man."

He leaned back in the chair and crossed one leg over the other.

"What made it such a lucky thing's the setup. At first I couldn't believe how great it was that she'd go for a slob like me. But there's somethin' even better, somethin' that made me think maybe there really *is* a God up there.

"The long and the short of it, Doc, is this: she lives in my building. Imagine that, a beautiful woman who latches on to me, and she lives *in my building*. Jeez, how lucky can a guy get? It's like manna droppin' from heaven. It's a gift from the genie in the bottle."

He peered at me expectantly.

I nodded my head, appreciating the upside to this arrangement, but knowing Ralph was in the office because something about his relationship with Laurel was bothering him sufficiently to bring him to a shrink.

"And to make it sweeter, she doesn't want a commitment. She just loves havin' sex with me. It's like a dream come true. Right, Doc?"

I nodded again, waiting for the other shoe to drop.

"So what happens? We begin this thing . . . whatever you wanna call it. We start seein' each other like two, three times a week. Maybe we go out for a quick bite somewhere and then we're back at her place; it's always her place—only two floors above mine. I gotta tell ya, Doc, it's the best sex I ever had in my life. It's just outta this world."

Ralph smiled, looked down at his hands, and shook his head.

"But after a few weeks, somethin' strange starts happenin'. After we make love, it's almost like some kinda spell comes over her. It's really weird. She goes into a trance or somethin'. Then she goes all wacko on me.

"She starts screamin' and slappin' me and throwin' things. First it was stuff like a pillow. Ya know, I thought it was some kinda game. But then it got serious. She threw an ashtray, nearly busted my head open. Then she began scratchin' me, and believe me, she has claws for fingernails."

Ralph described a series of postcoital attacks by Laurel—some more serious than others, but all pointing to one conclusion:

Laurel was a disturbed woman who, after sexual activity, entered into some altered state of consciousness during which violent impulses rose to the surface.

Ralph continued. "What really got me scared, and why I called the clinic, was what happened one night about a month ago. We go out for a bite and end up at her place. After we have sex, she gets that weird look in her eye, like she's in another world. I seen it before, and for sure I know she's gonna go nuts.

"This time she goes to the kitchen and comes out with a *knife*, a goddamned carving knife. Thing musta been a foot long. I almost shit my pants. I thought it was gonna be the end of me—that she'd stab me and it'd be all over. I grab her arm and pull the knife away, so she reaches for a lamp and hurls it at me. I just grabbed my pants and got the hell outta there before she ended up killin' me."

"Am I hearing you correctly?" I asked. "These attacks have gotten more serious?"

"You got it, Doc. She's been uppin' the ante."

"You said this happened nearly a month ago. So what's gone on since then?"

"Here's the thing, Doc, which is why I'm here." Ralph paused and again looked down at his hands. "As much as I tell myself it's nuts to go back there, I keep goin' back for more."

"So you've gone back since the knife incident?"

"I hate to admit it, but yeah, I've gone back." He shook his head, closed his eyes, and exhaled loudly.

"How many times?"

"I dunno. Maybe five, six times since then. I keep tellin' myself it's nuts to go back, but I just can't stop seein' her. And I gotta tell ya, Doc, I'm really gettin' worried."

"You should be. You're flirting with a very dangerous situation."

"I'm not just worried she'll hurt me . . . There's somethin' else."

"What's that?"

"I'm worried I'll end up hurtin' her."

I nodded, readily appreciating how these trysts with Laurel could become deadly. It was easy to imagine a catastrophic consequence in this scenario: while he was defending himself—or because of an adrenaline spike during a fight-or-flight response—one swipe of Ralph's bearlike arm could virtually decapitate Laurel. And those huge hands of his could clench into lunch-box-sized fists.

"Someone could get seriously hurt," I said.

"The last time she went for me, I end up shovin' her, and she flies across the room, bangs her head against the wall, slides down, and passes out. She's just lyin' there like a rag doll. I get really scared I mighta hurt her. I begin shakin' her, and thank God, she comes to."

"I think there's danger both ways," I said. "She could seriously hurt or even kill you, and on the other hand, you might end up hurting her."

"I know I can defend myself, Doc. What I really worry about is that I'll end up hurtin' her. Or maybe she'll call the cops. Or the neighbors might hear her screamin' at the top of her lungs and call 911." Ralph sighed so heavily, his chest heaved. "That's all I need—the cops come and arrest me on some domestic violence rap. And the next thing I know, I lose my PI license. Or my permit to carry gets suspended, maybe revoked. Then I'm outta business; I'm up the creek."

"So the sex comes with plenty of potential cost, doesn't it?"

"You got it, Doc. I gotta stop seeing her. I just gotta stop."

"Then why don't you?"

It was a naive question and I knew it. Ralph may have had some deep-seated need to court danger or maybe to engage in potentially self-defeating behavior—a wish to upset the relatively comfortable equilibrium of his life. I thought momentarily of asking about his early life, to learn if there was some long-standing pattern—a repetition compulsion—of self-injurious or destructive behavior. But I wasn't certain that would do much good at so critical a point in his relationship with Laurel.

"Hey, Doc, you're not gonna psychoanalyze me, are you?"

"Not at all," I said, knowing with complete certainty an excavation of Ralph's personality style and functioning couldn't be on the menu. Not in any realistic way. The problem may have stemmed from a riptide of underlying issues going back to childhood, but that could take forever to uncover. Even if he was willing to embark on a trek into his deepest psychological terrain, Ralph needed behavioral results—change—pronto, as quickly as possible.

"You're in a serious situation," I said, "and I think we should focus on how to get out of it, *soon.*"

"I know, Doc. The thing is . . . I keep goin' back there. I never had a woman who could lure me like this, who satisfies me like Laurel. I can't stay away. Don't get me wrong; I know the danger. I'm not stupid, but I just can't help myself. I keep goin' back for more."

"For more what?"

"For the sex and what it does for me."

"What does it do for you?"

"Makes me feel, I don't know . . ." He shook his head. "I can't describe it. It's just impossible to stay away. I mean, I know I could find sex in a hundred places, but somethin' about her drives me crazy. I can't stay away."

"Is there anything else she gives you, besides great sex?"

"Maybe, but I can't figure it out. Whatever it is, I can't stop myself. There's somethin' about her—her look, her body, even the way she smells—it keeps pullin' me back."

"So your common sense gets trampled by Laurel's sexual lure, right?"

"You got it, Doc. I gotta get my head straight—stay the hell away from her. There's too much on the line."

We set up a schedule of once-weekly appointments. The goal was simple: to help Ralph end this increasingly dangerous relationship.

After three more meetings, Ralph managed to cut down his visits to Laurel to once a week.

But he was unable to completely stop seeing her.

The dangerous cycle of sex and violence continued.

I kept pointing out to Ralph how his judgment became clouded—completely trumped—by his testosterone-poisoned urges. I heard myself repeating the same stale bromides about his primal needs blotting out his better judgment and how he was ignoring the potentially life-threatening and serious legal and financial consequences of this scenario.

But his willingness to deal with the danger of these hormonally driven liaisons fell victim to his urges.

At our sixth meeting, Ralph sported a patchwork of partly healed scratches on both cheeks. With a heavy sigh, he plopped down in the chair and then shook his head. His lips formed a tight line. His huge face sagged as we sat facing each other. His slumped posture oozed defeat.

He then launched into a description of yet another tryst with Laurel, which ended as did all the others. "So here I am again, Doc, sittin' across from you with egg on my face . . . or should I say with claw marks? And no matter what we say here, *I keep goin' back.*"

Sitting across from Ralph, I felt frustrated by my inability to help him. He certainly realized the dilemma in which he was snared. But having insight and being able to *act* on his self-knowledge were remarkably different accomplishments.

It was the old psychotherapy truth: insight about one's behavior doesn't guarantee a quick solution.

What could I say that might energize his readiness to change?

I'd run out of words.

Finally, Ralph said, "What am I doin', Doc? I know exactly what could happen and still I go back. Why?"

"Why do you think you go back?" I asked, groping for something to say—*anything* that could possibly make a difference.

"I don't know, damn it. Why can't I stop seeing her?"

The answer came to me out of nowhere.

"You can't stop because the penis has a short memory."

Ralph's mouth dropped; his eyes widened. His face reddened; he reared his huge head back and convulsed in an eruption of laughter.

He laughed so forcefully, his shoulders heaved. Tears formed in his eyes, and between chortles and snorts, he said, "'The penis has a short memory.' That's a good one, Doc."

His face was crimson. Nearly breathless and almost choking with laughter, he said, "I'm tryin' to picture that, a penis with a brain."

He snorted and laughed some more.

I don't know how truly funny my comment was, but Ralph's laughter was contagious. We both sat there, laughing at the preposterous analogy.

"'The penis has a short memory,'" Ralph repeated, still laughing. He wiped tears from his eyes.

Without realizing it would accomplish much, my off-the-cuff joke seemed to have hit Ralph right between the eyes.

It had meaning for him.

At the end of the session, still smiling, he got out of the chair, went to the office door, turned, and with a mallet-sized hand on the doorknob, said, "I'll remember that. 'The penis has a short memory.' Ha!"

He stepped out of the office and closed the door. His laughter resounded as he made his way down the clinic hallway.

A week later he returned for his next session.

"Well, Doc, I stayed away from her. I haven't been back."

He looked squarely at me.

"The penis has a short memory," he said, but this time, instead of gales of laughter, his tone was dead serious. It seemed as though the joke had been—for Ralph—some kind of astonishing revelation.

We talked about the week he'd spent since our last appointment. Oddly, we touched only lightly on the situation with Laurel. I had the feeling Ralph's psychological thermostat was changing, and the relationship with Laurel might change, too.

Sure enough, over the next three weeks he was barely tempted to resume the risky liaison, one that before then had held such powerful sway over him. He'd stayed away from Laurel even though she'd telephoned him a few times.

The following week he said Laurel was telephoning him more frequently.

"Hey, Doc. You know what I did yesterday?"

I looked at him questioningly, wondering if he'd succumbed to temptation once again.

"I called a real estate agency. I'm lookin' for another place. This Laurel thing's just too damned risky. I can't afford to take any more chances. I keep thinking about what you said . . . the penis has a short memory."

A few sessions later, we ended what could only be called a successful therapy. Ralph was moving out of his building—away from Laurel—and was moving on with his life.

Something was very clear: my wisecrack had been phrased in language that resonated deeply for Ralph. For whatever reason, it inspired the change he made—one that nothing said before that joke was capable of effecting.

I learned something from my brief interface with Ralph, a

principle that's guided me in dealing with patients ever since.

As a therapist you need to be different with different patients. What works with one person may fail dismally with another. The complexities of the human mind notwithstanding, and despite the labyrinthine guidelines for doing psychotherapy, a behavior-changing interpretation may be something as simple as a casual utterance that speaks directly to a patient's head, heart, and soul.

It may even be nothing more than a well-intended joke.

Afterword

I never heard from Ralph again.

I assume he went on with his life the best way he could. Perhaps he fell into similar situations farther down the road; perhaps not.

I'll never know.

Ralph and his treatment have stayed in my mind for years.

Here are the reasons:

For a very long time mental health professionals have debated the effectiveness of psychotherapy as a tool for healing and change.

Some take a biological approach, claiming medication is the most effective way to treat various problems and bring about behavioral change.

Others feel psychotherapy is crucial, either with or without medication. In that camp, some clinicians argue the relationship between therapist and patient is the most important element of the treatment process. Some even feel medication has no more than a placebo effect, stressing the inherent powers of belief in ridding patients of symptoms and difficulties.

In my view, there are elements of truth in all these positions. There are no clear-cut answers or simple formulas when dealing with the vast and virtually incomprehensible complexities of the human mind.

Over the years I've employed psychotherapy with some patients. With others I've taken a more medication-oriented approach. At times I've used a combination of both. I've tried my best to use whatever seemed appropriate for a particular person at a given time in his or her life.

For Ralph, medication would have been completely ineffective. Goal-specific, short-term psychotherapy seemed to have its limits until that one "joke" of an interpretation was made. It hit home with Ralph in a way nothing else before it had been able to do.

It may have been the power of common sense combined with humor. It may have been those two elements in the context of a good *relationship* that turned the tables on Ralph's risky and self-destructive behavior. It may have been no more than his belief in the power of those words, much akin to the powerful beliefs of primitive people in the healing powers of tribal shamans.

It may have been all or none of these factors.

I really have no idea what precisely made the difference for him.

But in the end Ralph was freed from his compulsion.

And that was the best outcome I could ever have hoped for.

A Deeper Cut

It began with a phone call from the Department of Surgery. Joe Sebold, a young attending surgeon with whom I'd gone to medical school, was on the line. We'd first met—literally—over a formalin-preserved cadaver on a steel dissecting table in the gross anatomy lab. We'd stayed in touch ever since. Joe and I hadn't crossed paths for some months, so we exchanged a few pleasantries, catching up on hospital gossip and each other's lives.

"We have a patient on the ward I'd really like you to see," Joe said.

"What's going on?"

"Her name's Mary C. She's a forty-year-old woman who, for all intents and purposes, lives on the surgery ward. Every time we discharge her, it's only a few weeks before she ends up right back here. She's had ten hospital admissions over the last three years. Her chart's probably two feet thick.

"She comes in with one kind of pain or another—usually in the abdomen. But it's not limited to that. She complains of dizziness, weakness, problems breathing, and fatigue. Some of this seems minor; some sounds serious. But it's always the same: no matter how much we work her up, we can't find anything wrong. Every test is normal—the lab work, all the X-rays and scans, you name it. I'm convinced it's in her head, that nothing's physically wrong with her."

"You think she's faking?"

"No. I think she actually experiences pain," he speculated.

"It's most likely psychogenic pain."

"That's how I look at it. Hey, you know the routine. If you come to the hospital enough times and complain about pain, eventually the surgeons'll open you up. You know us . . . We're always looking to cut. Remember the old joke from gross anatomy? *When in doubt, cut it out.* She's had so many organs removed, she has a checkerboard abdomen."

Joe was referring to a patient who'd undergone so many surgical procedures, her abdomen was crisscrossed with scars. In quasi-medical parlance, it was labeled a checkerboard abdomen. In those days there were no MRIs. Sophisticated tests and laparoscopic procedures hadn't been fully developed. If you came to the hospital frequently and complained of abdominal pain, surgeons would eventually do an exploratory laparotomy—they'd open you up and search inside, looking for something wrong. The biggest problem was that so many abdominal surgeries could cause adhesions to form around the intestines. They could cause pain and even obstruction, leading to yet more surgeries.

"I'm no Freudian type," Joe said, "but I'm positive there's something psychological going on with Mary—and whatever it is, it keeps her coming back. She's been on the ward for four days, and we haven't found a thing wrong, other than abdominal adhesions. The senior attending thinks we might have to take another look inside. I'm seriously thinking she has Munchausen syndrome."

Munchausen syndrome is a label applied when a patient either exaggerates or purposely *creates* medical signs and symptoms— for example, even going so far as rubbing a thermometer against a blanket to cause the mercury to shoot to a feverish level. The feigning of medical illness is done to gain attention, sympathy, or comfort. The end result: elaborate, costly medical workups with no diagnosable condition found.

Sometimes called "hospital hoppers," these people find comfort in the role of patient, being looked after by the staff. It seems to fill some deeply held, unresolved psychological need, most likely from childhood.

"I think she needs help," Joe said. "And whatever it is, another surgery isn't the answer."

When I arrived, the women's surgical ward was a maelstrom of activity, with nurses and aides tending to a full house of patients.

At the nursing station, I introduced myself as the attending psychiatrist who'd been asked to see Mary C. At the mention of the patient's name, the nurse shot me a glance that said, *She needs you more than a surgeon.*

I pored through Mary C.'s voluminous chart. Every conceivable test in the medical arsenal had been done—every bodily fluid had been analyzed; every possible radiologic procedure had been performed. And, as Joe had said, she'd undergone a host of exploratory and other surgeries over the course of years. Except for a few minor things—including not-so-minor intestinal adhesions—no objective indication of significant disease had ever been found. She was a diagnostic conundrum.

I made my way down the hallway and knocked on the door to her room.

A private room in Manhattan Hospital. A rare situation.

"Come in," a thin voice called.

Mary C. was lying comfortably in bed. There were no IV tubes or other medical paraphernalia—no monitors beeping, and none of the usual equipment seen in pre- or post-op patients' rooms. The head of the bed was elevated.

She wore a blue hospital gown and had short, reddish brown hair, fair skin, and green eyes. She was a thin—almost wispy-looking—woman. Her lips spread into a smile when I approached and introduced myself.

"Dr. Joe told me you'd be coming," she said, crossing her arms over her chest. "I don't need to be psychoanalyzed."

She was calling Joe Sebold by his first name. Her frequent hospital visits had bred a level of familiarity with the surgical staff. She was probably on a first-name basis with most of the ward personnel.

"I won't psychoanalyze you," I said, pulling a chair over to the bedside. "Dr. Joe just asked me to see how you're doing. He's worried about you."

"Oh, there's nothing to worry about," she said. "Except for Dr. Joe and the nurses, nobody talks to me around here. Everyone's in a rush. The doctors make short shrift of me. They don't think there's anything wrong."

"Well, I'm not rushing anywhere, so maybe we can talk for a while."

"That's fine," she said with another smile. She pressed a button, bringing the head of the bed to a more upright position.

"I see you have a room all to yourself."

She nodded. "It's the isolation room. I have it for the time being. If someone needs isolation, I'll move to another one."

"I understand you've been here a few times . . ."

"Oh yes," she said with a hint of a smile. "They'll start charging me rent soon."

"So what's brought you here this time?"

She sighed. "I've been tired and dizzy, and I've had trouble breathing. I just can't catch my breath. But the worst thing's this pain. Right here," she said, pointing to the middle of her abdomen. "It's been terrible. It makes me nauseous, and I've lost weight, maybe five pounds over the last few weeks. And I've been throwing up, too."

"I know you've had lots of trouble over the years. Have you been sick much in your life?"

"When I was a kid, I was sick all the time. I had lots of strep throats and swollen glands. I had my tonsils and adenoids taken out when I was twelve. And I always had trouble breathing. When I was five or six, the doctor said I probably had asthma. They don't think I have it now, but I still have trouble breathing. Sometimes I get so short of breath I feel like fainting. That's been going on for years."

I wondered if she was actually describing anxiety—hyperventilating and blowing off oxygen to the point where she would grow faint. Light-headedness was one of the most common complaints among patients experiencing episodes of anxiety or incipient panic attacks.

"In high school I had an elevator pass because I couldn't climb stairs without fainting. In my third year of high school I had my appendix taken out. If it isn't one thing, it's another," she said with a sigh. "And now the doctors think I have a heart murmur, too. But they said it's very mild, that maybe ten percent of people have it; so it's not a big thing."

So it was a well-entrenched pattern of lifelong sickness for Mary C. It would be difficult—nearly impossible—to break this enduring self-perception.

"I understand you've had a number of surgeries."

"Well, I always had cramps and plenty of trouble with my periods. They did lots of scrapings but didn't find anything. But it kept up—the pain and cramps—so they operated and found a cyst on my ovary. I had that removed.

"And I told you about the appendix operation; they thought it might rupture and I'd get. . . what do you call it, peritonitis? But they said the appendix looked normal when they took it out." The skin around her eyes tightened. "There was my gallbladder and some others.

"You know what?" she said. "I can't even remember them all. It's been so many things. There was something going on with my bladder, but that went away. And then there's been the whole thing with my uterus. They thought it was fibroids but couldn't find anything. Eventually I had a complete hysterectomy. I had my tubes and ovaries removed, too. There were others—I can't remember how many—where they opened me up to see what was going on, but they couldn't find a thing. It's been very frustrating."

"What's been frustrating?"

"That I'm in constant pain and they can't find anything." She paused for a moment. "Oh, they did find adhesions in my intestines. The doctors said I'd had so many surgeries that adhesions formed, and they can cause pain, even an obstruction. I had a few operations for them."

I realized letting Mary C. ramble on without directing the interview would result in her offering little more than a litany of physical complaints along with an encyclopedic history of surgeries, tests, procedures, and hospital admissions. Our talk could end up feeding her need to focus on bodily sensations and complaints. But it was a surefire way of establishing some rapport with her—she was obviously comfortable talking about her physical problems.

"This time I've been here for four days and they haven't found a thing wrong with me. I'm in constant pain and they don't know why. It's the same old thing.

"One of the doctors said I'd need more testing—some kind of blood test. I can't remember the name of it. And maybe some more scans because I feel weak and I have trouble breathing. But I'm not anemic and the pulmonary tests are normal." She sighed. "I don't know what's next, and the doctors don't either."

"Tell me about your family," I said, trying to deflect the cascade of medical details.

"I'm alone now. I have nobody who's really . . ." She stopped midsentence and shook her head.

"What just happened?" I asked.

"Well, there was a man once. He and I had this thing going, and I got pregnant but I lost the baby. He took off after that."

"When was that?"

"Oh, about twenty years ago."

"Has there been anyone since then?"

"Nope, not really." She had a faraway look in her eyes. "And I have a brother and sister."

"Where do you fit in, age-wise?"

"I'm the oldest."

"Tell me a little about yourself, your childhood."

"There isn't too much to tell," she began, pulling herself to a more upright position. "My father died when I was ten and Mom took care of everything. She worked as a cashier."

"Since you were the oldest, did some responsibilities fall on your shoulders?"

"Not really. I had trouble breathing, was always getting sick, you know? Just like what's happening now." She laughed softly. "Yeah, I'm the oldest, but because of my condition, everyone joked about it . . ."

"Joked about what?"

"That I was the oldest, but the sickest. Mom even called me the baby of the house. I didn't like that."

"That she called you the baby?"

"Yeah. It was . . . I don't know; it made me feel bad."

"How about your brother and sister? How'd they treat you?"

"They were good kids. And they were good to me. My brother's an insurance agent and lives in California. My sister's down in Florida with her husband and their two kids. I see them maybe once every year or two. But I really can't travel anymore because of my breathing problems and the weakness. If I get on a plane . . . forget it."

"Is your mother still alive?"

"She's in a nursing home." Mary's chin trembled. "She has emphysema from smoking all her life. And she has some kind of dementia. The doctors aren't sure if it's Alzheimer's or something else."

"So you really are alone, aren't you?"

"It's just me now, living here in New York." That faraway look returned to her eyes. "There were four of us, you know . . . ?"

"You, your brother, sister, and mother."

"No, I mean four kids."

"Four of you?"

"Yes. I was a twin."

She fell silent, blinking a few times. Her eyes looked unfocused. "You *were* a twin . . ."

More silence. Then she said, "She's dead."

"When did she die?"

"She died when we were five—leukemia."

More silence. She looked away, as though riveted on some distant object.

My thoughts swirled. A twin. Dead. She used the word *we*. *"She died when we were five."*

Twinship—one of the most powerful bonds possible between human beings.

"Do you remember anything about that?"

She nodded, still looking away. It seemed she was no longer in the hospital room talking with me.

A few moments passed before she turned to me and said, "Oh, yes, I remember her. She was very sick for a few months." Her voice trembled. "I definitely remember it. She went to the hospital for tests and treatment, and finally she went and . . . and she never came back."

Tears shivered on Mary's lower eyelids. She dabbed at them with her index finger.

I waited, hoping she would say something indicating an awareness of the emotional pull of her twin sister's death. But she remained silent.

Finally I said, "What's making you cry?"

She shook her head. "I don't know. It was a long time ago, and I only remember a little bit about her. After all, we were only five when she died."

"But you remember her."

She nodded.

Would she process the meaning of her twin sister's death in the trajectory of her own life?

"We were identical twins. I remember Mom saying we were two peas in a pod."

"Do you remember anything else about her?"

More tears formed at the corners of her eyes and then slid down over her cheekbones. "I don't know," she said. "Maybe it's an old wives' tale . . ."

I waited, but she remained silent. I'd long before learned when a patient devalued a remark by prefacing it with an utterance such as *Maybe it's an old wives' tale*, or *I know it's ridiculous, but . . .* a statement of great personal significance would follow. It was almost an unwritten law of the unconscious mind.

But she remained silent.

"What old wives' tale were you about to tell me?"

She sighed once again and whispered, "My mother always told me when it came to getting sick—even something like a cold or a sore throat—I'd always seem to get double the amount." She closed her eyes. "She said one twin would always get enough for the both of them. That was what the doctor always told her."

"You mean *after* your sister died?"

She nodded and looked away.

"So when you got sick, you were really twice as sick as anybody else would be?"

She sobbed. "I never really thought about it, but now that you ask, I remember my mother saying that."

"Saying what?"

"That I'd get sick enough for two . . . not just myself, but for the two of us."

"Why do you think she said that?"

"Who knows? But it's funny . . . There wasn't really any serious illness in the family that I can remember. The other kids were all pretty healthy."

She'd deflected my question.

"But *you* had a lot of illnesses," I said.

"If it wasn't me, it could have been somebody else."

Somebody else? The answer seemed obvious.

"You just said, 'If it wasn't me, it could have been somebody else.' Who else could it have been?"

"Well, if I wasn't the one always getting sick, it would have been my sister or brother."

"Maybe if your twin sister had lived, *she'd* have had half the sickness you've had all these years?"

"Who knows? It could've been my brother or my sister in Florida. But I wouldn't wish this on them. I mean the aches and pains, the problems breathing, the weakness, and the cramps . . . the gallbladder, my appendix, and all the hospitalizations, the tests and whatnot . . . I'd never want it to happen to either of them."

She'd backpedaled from the notion of guilt about surviving her twin sister—her alter ego. Yes, she'd resorted to an outpouring of medical minutiae. It confirmed my thought about her having survived.

I forced myself to refrain from pushing, from forcing her to talk about her dead twin sister. It would be too great a challenge for her to struggle with the notion of her survivorship. Could she ever grapple with the idea of something occurring when she was five years old having had such a profound impact on her for the next thirty-five years?

We spent more time talking. She commented in exquisite detail about the hospital, the food, the nurses, and other staff members. It was clear she'd formed good relationships with nearly everyone, but it was a different story when it came to the doctors.

"You know, you're the only doctor other than Dr. Joe who actually sat down and talked with me. The nurses here are great. They're like sisters to me . . ."

"*Sisters?*"

She nodded. "But the doctors? It's all rush-rush with them. When they ask 'How're you doing today?' they have one foot out the door. They're in and out of here in a flash. I think they're annoyed with me, but you actually sat down and talked with me."

"You mentioned the doctors are annoyed with you. Do you think they're frustrated by you?"

"I think so. I can't say I blame them. They can't figure out what's wrong."

"Well, why do you think Dr. Sebold asked me to see you?"

"He doesn't think I'm crazy, does he?" She laughed, but uncertainty seeped through her voice.

"He doesn't think that at all."

"I'm just so frustrated by all this—the tests and surgeries—and I'm still the same."

"I think Dr. Sebold's frustrated, too," I said.

"Meanwhile, I can't get over this." She sighed.

"Can't get over what?"

"I can't get rid of the aches and pains, the cramps, the breathing problems, the fatigue, and all this dizziness. It's such a burden."

"I'm sure it is," I said, knowing our time together was drawing to an end. "Would you like to talk with someone? Maybe get some counseling about how to deal with your frustration?"

She shook her head. "I like talking with you. I really do," she said, nodding her head while looking directly at me. "But I don't need any psychological help. I need help with my . . ." She paused, seemingly lost in thought.

"You need help with what?" I asked, knowing full well what her reply would be.

"With whatever's going on in my body. I need the doctors to find out what the hell's wrong and just fix it, once and for all."

"Okay, I understand," I said, standing up. "But why don't you give it some thought. Maybe talking with someone will help."

"I'll think about it."

I called Joe Sebold twice over the next two days, but he was tied up with surgeries and conferences.

There was no rush to speak with him since Mary would be on the ward for a few more days. If I'd heard her correctly, more tests were on the horizon, but with the weekend approaching, they wouldn't be scheduled until at least Monday.

While I couldn't be terribly optimistic—after all, this deeply ingrained pattern had been ongoing for years—I decided to tell Joe there was a *chance*, however slight, that Mary might agree to getting some counseling at our clinic.

But I was a young psychiatrist then and hadn't yet come to terms with the notion that people sometimes needed their repetitive behaviors—their defensive crusts—to protect themselves from deeper, more painful truths about themselves and their lives.

I decided I'd tell Joe that Mary's never-ending pattern of hospital stays had deep meaning for her. I would say that Mary's coming to the hospital so often was an encapsulation of much of her life. I'd tell him what I'd learned about her by sitting down and talking with her, by listening to her. I would clue him in on her twin's death and its life-altering repercussions.

I'd tell him about the power of twinship in identical twins—how they could feel they're virtually one and the same person. After all, they share identical DNA. And parents often dress them alike and emphasize the twinship in so many ways, as do relatives, friends, and everyone else in their lives. The idea of being one and the same person infiltrates twins' beings. The bond can be so powerful, identical twins may have trouble differentiating themselves from each other.

I would tell Joe about the tragedy of Mary's life: her identical twin sister's death at age five had triggered a lifelong commitment to illness in her own life.

I would tell Joe that Mary suffered from survivor's guilt. Her need to feel sick and check herself into the hospital—again and again—wasn't a willful attempt to gain attention or succor from the staff.

No, it wasn't Munchausen syndrome at all.

Rather, it was her way of seeking expiation for having lived while her twin sister died. To put it another way: she was taking on a double dose of illness.

She'd been doing it for nearly thirty-five years.

The chance Mary would benefit from counseling seemed slim. But it wouldn't hurt to try weaning her away from an unending carousel of hospitalizations and surgeries.

Maybe she could form a good relationship with a therapist—a woman resident in Manhattan Hospital's psychiatric outpatient clinic—with whom she might bond strongly, and to whom she could relate, instead of seeking out endless bouts of surgery.

Who could know if it would do any good for her?

But it was worth a try. I hated the notion of giving up on hope.

Two days later Joe got back to me.

"You won't believe what happened," he said.

"What?"

"Mary got worse. She was in agony with abdominal cramps. It got so bad, she was screaming in pain. So the senior attending surgeon decided to open her up again. He didn't think it was the adhesions because she wasn't obstructed and wasn't vomiting. He thought we'd find a lesion in her pancreas. So we operated. There was no obstruction; the pancreas and everything else was completely normal."

"So the beat goes on," I said.

"Not anymore. While she was on the table, she went into cardiac arrest and died. It was a reaction to the anesthesia. The autopsy was negative for any pathology, just some old adhesions from the surgeries."

Mary C. had finally joined her twin sister.

The power of the mind would never stop amazing me.

Afterword

Mary C.'s tragedy is emblematic of the enduring power of twinship.

It also highlights an important issue in the practice of general medicine. Conservative estimates indicate that 5 percent of people presenting in doctors' offices suffer from psychogenic symptoms—these include pain, neurologic and gastrointestinal complaints, and sexual difficulties—none of which have any physical basis. In other words, underlying these patients' physical symptoms are psychiatric problems.

These difficulties are generally known as psychosomatic or somatoform disorders, situations in which mental and emotional conflicts cause *bodily* symptoms that cannot be traced to any physical cause.

As was the case with Mary C., people with these disorders are not faking their symptoms. The pain and discomfort they experience are real and can affect daily functioning, sometimes to a severe degree.

Before a somatoform disorder can be diagnosed, tests must be done to rule out any possible physical causes for a patient's complaints. Unfortunately, these tests and procedures by their very nature *reinforce* the notion of physical illness in the person's mind. When testing is negative for physical pathology, these patients are often dissatisfied by a lack of explanation for their symptoms and visit other doctors, seeking answers. This scenario ends up creating a cycle of medical tests and "doctor shopping," often persisting for years. The enduring quest for medical answers and explanations may lead to a great deal of anxiety. Complicating matters, physicians often feel pressured to "do something" and end up prescribing medications for disorders existing only in the mind, thereby further reinforcing the notion of physical pathology.

The most well-known of the somatoform disorders is hypochondriasis. Someone with this ailment is intensely preoccupied by the notion of having a serious disease and believes minor bodily sensations are signs of significant illness. The patient may think nausea is an indication of stomach cancer or a headache signals a brain tumor.

"No one understands what I'm going through" is a frequent lament of someone suffering from hypochondriasis.

The ongoing series of complaints about not feeling well often frustrates and then drives away family and friends. The resulting isolation deepens the person's focus on the phantom illness.

Somatoform disorders are long-standing, deeply entrenched conditions. They're generally refractory to treatment by internists, family practitioners, or psychiatrists. In the service of shielding the self from an unacceptable or frightening psychological reality, the hypochondriac's mind redirects its focus away from emotional conflict to the body and its physical sensations.

This maladaptive pattern begins years before anyone can see it for what it truly is.

Remember Mary C.'s frequent childhood illnesses and breathing difficulties. Could a parent or doctor have been expected to perceive her maladies for what they actually were? So, beginning soon after her sister's death, continuing in adolescence and through adulthood, Mary's mind redirected guilt and anguish over her twin's untimely death onto a constellation of bodily sensations.

Mary felt physical pain, but its source wasn't a gallbladder, a uterus, or an ovary; rather, it was her mind attempting to deal with the meaning of her sister's death in the only way it knew: redirection. And that coping mechanism had entrenched itself deeply over thirty-five years.

Had Mary C. lived, it's doubtful she would have accepted the notion that the root cause of her pain and discomfort was psychological. Indeed, most patients with somatoform disorders reject this idea and seek out other medical opinions.

Despite chronic physical pain and discomfort, these patients find it more tolerable to believe they are physically ill than to accept the premise that their entire way of life is compromised and in need of help.

In a very real way, for someone like Mary C., endless doctor shopping, medical tests, hospital visits, and surgeries can be understood as a sign of a deeper conflict, one that's unacceptable to the person's conscious mind. And that inner reality drives the behavior onward, again and again.

Having seen firsthand the very real suffering somatoform patients endure, and having been largely frustrated in my attempts to help them, I find the old joke about the inscription on the hypochondriac's tombstone, "See, I told you I was sick," to be profoundly sad and yet true.

A Brief Last Word

Throughout history and continuing today, mental illness has been stigmatized. The reason is clear: unlike physical illness with signs and symptoms such as pain, fever, bleeding, and shortness of breath, mental illness often presents with *unacceptable and disturbing behaviors.*

Whether it's the profoundly depressed, nearly catatonic patient, the raging psychotic, or someone suffering from uncontrollable anxiety or panic, the patient's aberrant behaviors elicit worry, fear, and revulsion in others.

In the early centuries of civilization, mental illness was thought to be caused by malevolent deities or astrological forces. During the Middle Ages, psychotic people were locked away in "madmen's towers" and were often forcibly expelled from towns and cities. By the fifteenth century, supernatural forces and witchcraft were believed to cause mental illness. Those afflicted were thought to be "possessed" by demons and underwent exorcism or torture, or were even killed.

For centuries places have been set aside to house the mentally ill. They were often referred to as asylums.

Traditionally, *asylum* (derived from Greek, Latin, and Late-Middle English) meant an institution for the maintenance and care of the mentally ill or other persons requiring specialized assistance. It defined an inviolable refuge or a secure retreat, a sanctuary.

But the unsavory view of mental illness created by fear, super-stition, and lack of knowledge perverted the perception of the asylum, away from being a safe haven to a strange place of unbri-dled madness.

Unfortunately, the stigma remains today.

He was taken to the nuthouse.

She belongs in an insane asylum.

He was carted off to the loony bin.

These expressions are examples of that distorted view. Paren-thetically, the word *loony* derives from *lunar*, meaning *moon*. This reflects the centuries-old belief that a full moon causes an upsurge in madness—otherwise known as *lunacy* and giving rise to the word *lunatic*.

Society's treatment of the mentally ill is a long and tragic saga. Often referred to as *inmates* rather than patients, this term is emblematic of people's views of mental illness. During the eigh-teenth century, so-called inmates of European mental asylums were regarded as suffering from incurable conditions. They were subjected to torture, physical restraints, frequent beatings, and years of forced incarceration, deepening the tainted image of the institutions housing them.

By the second half of the twentieth century—during the late 1940s and early 1950s—many chronically psychotic patients were hospitalized and subjected to lobotomies. In this surgery, the white matter of the brain's frontal lobes was destroyed, resulting in marked changes and deterioration of patients' personalities. Fortunately, by the late 1950s, with the advent of new and effective medications, lobotomies virtually disappeared as a "therapeutic" tool.

The stigmatization of mental illness and psychiatric hospital-ization continues to this day.

Of the many criticisms hurled at psychiatry as a medical spe-cialty, perhaps the most biting one is a misconception that it has not changed significantly for the last sixty years.

This belief is not true.

Over the last few decades, the treatment of psychiatric patients has advanced dramatically.

Extremely effective medications have been developed, including potent antipsychotic remedies, effective antidepressants, antianxiety medications, and mood stabilizers.

Innovative treatments have evolved, including light therapy, transcranial magnetic stimulation, sophisticated neuroimaging, and more advanced techniques for administering electroconvulsive therapy.

More are on the way.

Psychiatry and medicine are now on the cusp of revolutionary new developments. These include the potential for gene therapy and the discovery of new biological markers for many illnesses. Neurocognitive and neurobiological markers for schizophrenia, bipolar disorder, and other major psychiatric conditions have been discovered. These advances implicate specific brain pathways and chemical neurotransmitters as playing crucial roles in various forms of psychopathology. Neuroimaging of the brain has evolved whereby specific structural abnormalities are observed and monitored for some psychiatric illnesses.

Certain *predictive* drug-related biomarkers will soon be used to indicate whether a particular medication will be effective for an individual.

In the not-too-distant future biomarkers will likely make it possible to *prevent* the onset of mental illness and will be used to individually tailor treatments for those already affected.

Equally important, these new developments do not discount the benefits patients may derive from psychotherapy. In fact, for psychotherapy to be effective, it must work through biological mechanisms. Many neuroimaging studies have demonstrated that psychotherapy can affect the brain as profoundly as medication, electroconvulsive therapy, and deep brain stimulation.

Over the last sixty years more advances have been made in understanding and treating mental illness than in all the centuries during which human beings have populated the earth. Even newer developments will change nearly everything about psychiatric treatment. Psychiatry as a medical specialty has entered the realm of neuroscience and is no longer viewed as a social science or the handmaiden of medicine. While enormous progress has been made, there is still much more to be accomplished.

Hopefully, these stories have shed light on psychiatry's attempts—not always successful—to bring relief to those suffering from mental illness. I hope they've also described some of the prevailing controversies in psychiatry: those concerning diagnosis, treatment options, deinstitutionalization, patient care, doctor-patient communication, confidentiality, medical malpractice, and forensic issues.

In the preface I mentioned a certain unity conveyed by this tapestry of stories. I hope these tales have, among other things, demonstrated that beneath the strange signs and symptoms of many mental disorders, deeper meaning can be found. As bizarre and inexplicable as some patients may appear, each one's unique life story has funneled down through the final common pathway of psychiatric illness. Most of them can be explained, if attention is paid.

Twenty years from now a psychiatrist writing a book similar to this one will very likely have many encouraging tales to tell.

I believe the future is bright, and there are ample reasons to be hopeful.

Glossary

This glossary is by no means a complete list of psychiatric/ medical terminology. Rather, it explains in a bit more detail some of the terms arising during the course of the stories told in this book.

adhesion. A band of scar tissue binding two organs or segments of organs that are not normally joined together. Adhesions may appear as thin sheets of tissue, or as thick fibrous bands. Adhesions may develop when the body's repair mechanisms respond to any tissue disturbance, such as surgery, infection, trauma, or radiation. Although adhesions can occur anywhere in the body, the area most commonly affected is the abdomen. Adhesions become surgical emergencies when they encircle the intestinal tract, causing bowel obstruction. (See "A Deeper Cut.")

Bedlam. The nickname for London's Bethlehem Royal Hospital, Europe's first institution for the treatment of mentally ill people. The word *bedlam*, meaning *uproar and confusion*, was a play on words when applied to the Bethlehem facility. Although the hospital became a modern psychiatric institution, historically it came to represent the worst excesses of that era with its inhuman treatment of patients. (See "King of the Puerto Ricans.")

bereavement. A normal and expectable reaction following the death of a loved one. It's a process involving grief, sadness, and a profound yearning for the deceased person. It may be colored by a pervasive sense of emptiness, but in contrast to depression, the bereaved person's self-esteem remains intact. A bereaved person does not suffer from profound feelings of self-loathing or guilt that characterize the depressed person's state of mind. There may be instances of *pathological* or *complicated* bereavement in which the bereaved person's mourning process is deepened by elements of depression or another form of pathology. Patricia A.'s bereavement became complicated by severe depression and elements of post-traumatic stress disorder. (See "Baptism by Fire.")

biological psychiatry. The branch of the specialty that views mental illness as being based on observable data only, such as physical findings and laboratory readings that quantify the disease process. This view posits that all psychiatric disorders are caused by one or a chain of measurable biochemical or physiological changes. This interpretation states any entity for which no biological basis can be found is not really a disease state. In this view the treatment for mental illness is strictly biologic and employs pharmacologic or physical methods only. (See "A Helping Hand.")

biomarkers. Short for "biological markers." Measurable indicators of the presence or severity of a disease, or a substance introduced to examine an organ's functioning. Biomarkers are characteristic substances detected and measured in blood or tissue. They may be specific cells, molecules, genes, gene products, enzymes, or hormones. Certain biomarkers are very well-known and have been used by physicians for years. For example, blood pressure is a biomarker used to determine the risk of stroke. Cholesterol levels are considered a biomarker and risk indicator for coronary and vascular disease, while C-reactive protein (CRP) is a biomarker for inflammation anywhere in the body.

Biomarkers have been most extensively used in the detection, screening, diagnosis, treatment, and monitoring of various cancers. New biomarkers are being discovered—not only for cancer but for a variety of physical and mental disorders. This very likely means someday it will be possible to determine the most effective therapeutic regimen for a specific mental disorder, and treatment will be individually and precisely tailored for a particular patient. (See "A Brief Last Word.")

bipolar disorder. Formerly called manic-depressive disorder. A serious mental illness characterized by periods of elevated mood alternating with episodes of depression. The heightened mood is known as mania or a *manic high*, which can be so severe the person is rendered psychotic. During a manic episode, the person feels inordinately happy, completely elated. There is an energetic, driven quality to the person, who may become irritable or even aggressive if confronted. Speech is pressured with flight of ideas, which involves rapid-fire sequences of random ideas with little connection to each other. Decisions are made with little or no thought of the consequences. An affected person has boundless energy and may not sleep for days at a time. The patient may go on a buying spree, spending enormous sums of money in an irresponsible way. (When I first saw Nathan B., I considered the possibility of his being in the throes of a manic high.)

I once treated a patient with bipolar disorder who, during a manic episode, spent a huge sum of money on furniture and expensive household goods. When the furniture was delivered, it could not fit through the apartment door. She then called a contractor to widen the doorway. Her family recognized the seriousness of her illness and had her hospitalized.

Between manic episodes there are periods of depression with all the hallmarks of major depression. There is a great risk of suicide during this phase of the disorder. (See **depression**.)

brachial plexus. A network of nerves running from the spine, proceeding through the neck, the armpit region, and into the arm.

The network supplies nerves to the skin and muscles of the upper arm, forearm, and hand. Phil M. sustained a permanent injury to his brachial plexus, one that changed the course of his life, causing him to be in near-constant pain, resulting in depression severe enough to require hospitalization. (See "Saved by a Cup of Joe.")

camisole. Also called a straitjacket. A garment shaped like a jacket with overlong sleeves, typically used to restrain a person who may otherwise cause harm to the self or others. Once the arms are inserted into the straitjacket's sleeves, they are then crossed over the chest. The ends of the sleeves are tied to the back of the wearer, ensuring that the arms are kept close to the chest with as little movement as possible. (See "Off the Wall.")

cardiac arrest. Also known as cardiopulmonary or circulatory arrest. The sudden stoppage of blood circulation due to the inability of the heart to contract effectively, or at all. Arrested blood circulation prevents delivery of oxygen and glucose to the body. Lack of oxygen and glucose to the brain causes loss of consciousness, which then results in abnormal or absent breathing. Brain injury is likely to happen if cardiac arrest goes untreated for more than five minutes. A cardiac arrest is different from (but may be caused by) a heart attack, where blood flow to the muscle of the heart is impaired. It is different from congestive heart failure, where circulation is substandard, but the heart is still pumping sufficient blood to sustain life. Patricia A.'s husband died of a sudden cardiac arrest after working out in a gym. (See "Baptism by Fire.")

catatonia. A condition marked by changes in muscle tone or activity associated with some serious mental and physical illnesses. In catatonic stupor the person experiences very little motor activity, remaining motionless. Catatonic excitement, or excessive movement, is associated with violent behavior directed toward one's self or others.

Catatonia can be present in patients suffering from physical and emotional conditions such as drug intoxication, depression, and schizophrenia. It is sometimes seen in severe mood disorders such as major depression. (See "Baptism by Fire.")

command hallucinations. Auditory hallucinations in which the person hears a voice, or voices, commanding certain actions to be taken. These are considered the most dangerous hallucinations because they often result in the affected person obeying the voice(s), thus taking action that may be harmful to the self or others. Many people with severe mental illness such as schizophrenia hear voices telling them to harm themselves or take actions harming others. Willie Mae E. experienced command hallucinations telling her to kill herself. In response to the voices, she jumped in the path of an oncoming train. Unlike many patients experiencing command hallucinations, Willie Mae was frightened by them and sought help. (See "When a Patient Knows More Than the Doctor.")

community ward. Sometimes called an open ward. A psychiatric unit that does not house acutely suicidal or homicidal patients. The focus in such a unit is to make life as normal as possible for patients, while continuing treatment to the point where they can be discharged. Patients are not allowed access to their own medications because of the risk of an impulsive overdose. Some open units are physically unlocked; others use locked entrances and exits, depending on the type of patients admitted. (The ward where Phil M. spent time was an open/community ward, as was the ward where Ellen and Gloria were hospitalized in the story "A Helping Hand.")

delusion. A rigidly held belief with strong conviction despite incontrovertible evidence to the contrary. It is distinct from a belief based on false or incomplete information, confabulation, dogma, illusion, or misperception. It is not a belief generally shared by one's

cultural or religious group. Delusions typically occur in the context
of neurological or severe mental illness, although they are not tied
to any particular disease and have been found to occur in the context of many pathological states (both physical and mental).

Delusions come in various forms:

Persecutory delusions involve the false notion that one is being
persecuted, followed, or harassed by others. The imagined perse-
cutors may be the police, politicians, the FBI, the CIA, the KGB,
or other government agencies, or may be friends, family members, or people in general.

Delusions of love involve the belief that some famous person is
in love with the afflicted—a movie star or political figure, or some
other person of great standing. Occasionally, a patient may present with a combination of persecutory and grandiose delusions.
Delusional thinking is one of the major hallmarks of psychosis—
the loss of the ability to differentiate reality from fantasy.

Grandiose delusions are characterized by the delusional person believing he or she is some great figure like God, Jesus,
Moses, or another religious or historical person. (See "King of
the Puerto Ricans.")

depression. A state of lowered mood pervading a person's
thoughts, feelings, and behavior. People with a severely depressed
mood (major or clinical depression) feel sad, anxious, empty,
hopeless, helpless, worthless, guilty, irritable, or restless. They
may lose interest in activities that were once pleasurable; experience loss of appetite or overeat; have difficulty concentrating,
remembering details, or making decisions; and may contemplate,
attempt, or commit suicide. Insomnia, excessive sleeping, fatigue,
aches, pains, digestive problems, or reduced energy may also be
present. Some patients presenting with major depression become
psychotic, thinking they are the worst people on the face of the
earth. In their psychotic form of self-denigration, they may hear

voices (auditory hallucinations) condemning them and confirming their devalued self-image. (See "Baptism by Fire" and "Saved by a Cup of Joe.")

downward drift. A hypothesis about the relationship between chronic mental illness and a person's social class. This view maintains that mental illness causes one to have a downward drift in social class. According to this theory, lower social class does not cause the onset of a mental disorder; rather, a person's deteriorating mental health occurs first, which results in a drifting downward in social attainment and class. Some mental health professionals argue the opposite, saying lower social class contributes heavily to mental illness.

It's likely the observed downward drift often seen in chronic schizophrenia is due to a combination of factors. There can be little doubt people suffering from delusions and hallucinations experience social and occupational deterioration as they cannot function adequately in society. Furthermore, because of intermittent or no treatment (due to factors cited in the story of Dr. Boris Papalini), their illnesses continue unabated, resulting in well-entrenched maladaptive world views. Some experts have posited that untreated schizophrenia *itself*, over time, causes degradation of brain functioning due to the effects of aberrant brain chemistry noted in such a disorder.

electroconvulsive therapy (ECT). Formerly called shock treatments. A form of therapy reserved for the relatively rare instances of depression refractory to the wide array of potent antidepressant medications available today. The horrendous popular view of ECT was best illustrated in the 1975 film *One Flew Over the Cuckoo's Nest*. Today the procedure is far different from what was being used in the 1970s. Now electrodes are placed on the same side of the head. A short-acting anesthetic and muscle relaxant are given. The muscle relaxant prevents a seizure from occurring.

A brief pulse current is delivered, as opposed to the sine wave currents used years ago. Usually, a series of shocks is administered over a period of weeks.

The most common side effects of ECT are temporary confusion and memory loss. The period of confusion is short. The patient has no memory of the hours leading up to the shock (retrograde amnesia) and little or no memory for some hours afterward (anterograde amnesia). The mechanism by which ECT improves depression is still unknown. (See "A Brief Last Word.")

epidural hematoma. A collection of blood caused by arterial bleeding between the dura mater (the covering of the brain) and the inner surface of the skull. It is usually caused by trauma to the skull. Epidural hematomas may not show any signs of injury at first, but then develop quickly into severe signs like coma. If not treated quickly, an epidural hematoma is often fatal. (See "Off the Wall.")

Fishkill Correctional Facility. A medium-security prison that is part of New York State's prison system. It is located in the town of Fishkill, which is in Beacon, New York. Fishkill Correctional Facility was constructed in 1896. It began as the Matteawan State Hospital for the Criminally Insane. The facility also houses the Regional Medical Unit for southern New York's prisons. In 1998 the prison was expanded to hold one hundred maximum-security inmates. (See "Behind Bars.")

flight of ideas. A symptom seen in the manic phase of bipolar disorder. It involves a continuous flow of rapid speech jumping from one topic to another. Topics are only loosely associated with each other. The patient is highly distractible, with speech veering off into different directions. There is often a great deal of word play. In severe mania, speech may become so disorganized as to be incoherent.

forensic psychiatry. A subspecialty of psychiatry related to the interface between law and psychiatry.

In criminal matters, forensic psychiatrists work with courts in evaluating an individual's competency to stand trial and competency to represent one's self at trial, and in assessing defendants claiming mental disorders in relation to an "insanity defense." Forensic psychiatrists also render testimony at trials and in hearings pertaining to criminal matters.

In civil law, forensic psychiatrists are called upon to evaluate people's competency to execute a will, enter into a contract, discharge one's self from a hospital against medical advice, or engage in activities involving civil legal matters where competency is in question.

A forensic psychiatrist may also testify at trial about psychiatric damages resulting from an accident or about other civil matters in litigation, including psychiatric malpractice cases where a departure from standard and accepted psychiatric practice allegedly occurred, or in cases claiming psychiatric damages suffered by a patient-plaintiff as a result of medical malpractice by a physician in another specialty.

four-point restraints. Physical restraints are sometimes used for patients who become violent and dangerous because of psychiatric illnesses or an altered mental status. The use of physical restraints may be necessary for patients' protection and to protect others. The application of limb restraints on both arms and legs at once is known as using four-point restraints. The limb restraints are soft, padded cuffs applied to a patient to prevent the patient from causing harm to him/herself or to others. The cuffs are wrapped around the patient's wrists and ankles and then attached to the bed frame. Great care must be taken because highly agitated patients requiring such restraints can overheat, become dehydrated, and develop life-threatening electrolyte imbalance.

Therefore, four-point restraints are used rarely and only for short periods of time. When the patient calms down, the restraints are removed.

guilt. An unpleasant emotional experience that occurs when a person realizes, or believes—whether justified or not—that he or she has compromised valued standards of conduct, or has violated an internalized moral code of conduct. Guilt can be experienced in relation to actual conduct, or as a reaction to fantasized or imagined misdoings. Guilt is very different from shame. (Contrast **shame.**)

hallucination. A perception in the absence of any external stimulus. It has qualities of a real perception. Hallucinations are vivid, substantial, and to the affected person seem located in external, objective space. In other words, they seem completely *real*. Hallucinations can occur in any sensory modality—visual, auditory, gustatory (taste), olfactory (smell), and tactile (feelings in the body). There are certain normal hallucinations such as those experienced while dreaming and sometimes experienced when one is drifting off to sleep or in the act of awakening from a deep sleep. Willie Mae E. was suffering from auditory command hallucinations. Patricia A. heard her husband's voice and was responding to it. Hallucinations, along with delusional thinking, are the major hallmark of psychosis. (See "Baptism by Fire" and "When a Patient Knows More Than the Doctor.")

illusion. The misinterpretation of an external reality. For instance, mistaking a stick on a country trail for a snake, or thinking the undulating waves of heat on a distant road represent an oasis, are commonly seen illusions.

informed consent. Permission obtained from a patient to perform a specific test or medical procedure. Informed consent is required before invasive procedures are performed and before a patient is admitted to a research study. The procedure, surgery, or test is explained to the patient in terms he or she can understand and includes an explanation of the benefits and potential risks involved.

In a *forensic psychiatric examination*, the examinee must be told by the examiner why the interview is being conducted and what is entailed. The examinee must be told there is no doctor-patient relationship; there is no doctor-patient confidentiality; no treatment will be offered; no advice or recommendations will be made; and a written report will be generated and become part of the legal documents of record.

An evaluating psychiatrist or psychologist who does not make certain a plaintiff knows the nature and purpose of the examination is violating the ethical rules of the medicolegal interface.

When I examined Aaron J., it was clear he was fully informed of the reasons for the evaluation and knew a written report would be forwarded to the defense and the plaintiff, Aaron J. (See "Behind Bars.")

inguinal hernia. A condition in which a loop of intestine enters the inguinal canal. In a man, it can sometimes slide down the inguinal canal and fill the scrotal sac. An inguinal hernia is usually repaired surgically to prevent the herniated segment of intestine from becoming strangulated, gangrenous, or obstructive, thereby blocking passage of waste through the bowel. Of all hernias, 75 to 80 percent are inguinal hernias. Calvin W. had a slowly progressing inguinal hernia, which was repaired at Manhattan Hospital. (See "The Head Doctor.")

laparoscopic surgery. Also called minimally invasive surgery. A modern surgical technique in which operations are performed through small incisions (usually 0.5–1.5 centimeters) in the body. Such a technique avoids the need to open the body cavity to access the organ on which the surgery is performed. Laparoscopic procedures have changed the landscape of surgery, and patients can be discharged far earlier with much less discomfort than was previously the case.

laparotomy. A surgical incision between the ribs and the pelvis, which offers surgeons a complete view inside the entire abdominal cavity. For the most part, exploratory laparotomy has been replaced by CT scans, MRIs, and other radiologic diagnostic tools. Mary C. had undergone multiple laparotomies, which resulted in extensive scarring (a checkerboard abdomen) and multiple adhesions. (See "A Deeper Cut.")

liaison psychiatry. Also known as consultative psychiatry. The branch of psychiatry specializing in the interface between medicine and psychiatry, usually taking place in a hospital or medical setting. The role of the hospital-based liaison psychiatrist is to evaluate patients at the request of the treating medical or surgical staff. Typical situations in which a liaison psychiatric consultation is requested involve a patient acting strangely on a medical or surgical ward, a patient demanding to be discharged against medical advice (AMA), or one refusing to take prescribed medication while hospitalized. The psychiatrist is asked to assess the patient's competency to make such a medical decision. My interface with Calvin W. involved liaison psychiatry. (See "The Head Doctor.")

light therapy. Also known as phototherapy. A treatment for seasonal affective disorder (SAD), which is sometimes referred to as "winter blues." This type of depression is related to changes in seasons. Some scientists have noted many nontropical animals exhibit less activity during winter months in response to the reduction in available food, reduced sunlight, and the hardship of surviving in cold weather. Even animals that do not hibernate often show changes in behavior during winter. It has been posited that SAD represents a remnant of a hibernation response in some remote ancestor. Presumably, food was scarce during most of human prehistory, and a tendency toward low mood during the winter months would have been adaptive by reducing the need for caloric intake. The preponderance of women with SAD suggests the response may also somehow regulate reproduction. Symptoms usually begin in the fall and continue through the winter months as the hours of daylight lessen.

Bright-light therapy is an effective treatment for this condition. SAD is more common at northern latitudes such as Finland, where the rate of SAD is 9.5 percent. There is evidence that many patients with SAD have abnormal circadian rhythm, and bright-light treatment can correct this problem. (See "A Brief Last Word.")

mourning. See **bereavement.**

Munchausen syndrome. A psychiatric disorder in which a person feigns disease, illness, or psychological trauma to obtain attention, sympathy, or reassurance. True Munchausen syndrome fits within the subclass of factitious (contrived) disorders with predominantly physical symptoms, along with a history of recurrent hospitalizations, and dramatic, extremely improbable tales of medical illness. It was initially thought Mary C. presented with Munchausen syndrome, but she was more accurately diagnosed as suffering from somatoform disorder. (See "A Deeper Cut.")

nervous breakdown. Not a medical term nor the name of a specific mental illness. Though it seems to be used less frequently these days, it's a layperson's term to describe an overwhelmingly stressful situation causing someone to become temporarily unable to function in day-to-day life. It connotes an overload of life stressors leading to an incapacitating upsurge in anxiety or depression. *Nervous exhaustion* and *nervous fatigue* are synonymous terms used occasionally to indicate the same situation.

panic disorder. A condition that involves recurring panic attacks. The symptoms of panic attacks are sudden and intense feelings of diffuse and nameless terror, fear, or a state of utter apprehension, without the presence of actual danger in the environment. There are usually physical correlates to a severe panic attack; they may involve shortness of breath, intense sweating, rapid and irregular heartbeat, feelings of light-headedness, fainting, dizziness, feelings of heat, tingling around the mouth and in the extremities, feelings of coldness, a sense of unreality, or feeling one is outside one's own body (depersonalization) or that one's surroundings appear unfamiliar (derealization), along with an imminent sense of doom. The affected person may actually feel he or she is dying.

The symptoms of a panic attack usually happen suddenly, peak within a few minutes, and then subside. Some attacks may last longer or may occur in succession, making it difficult to determine when one attack ends and another begins.

The attacks may become so frightening, the affected person fears being alone or away from home and feels he or she must be in a "safe" place. In such a case, the person may develop *agoraphobia*, which is fear of being away from home or a "safe" place. He or she may become homebound. (The word *agoraphobia* comes from the Greek word *agora*, meaning *marketplace*, while *phobia* means *fear*.)

I once treated a patient suffering from panic disorder with agoraphobia so severe, she not only was afraid to leave her home but feared leaving her bedroom. She was literally bedroom-bound.

Her husband forcibly dragged her to my office. Medication along with supportive psychotherapy helped her eventually resume a normal life.

paranoia. A psychotic disorder characterized by intense feelings of suspicion and/or delusions of persecution with or without grandeur, often strenuously defended by the affected person with apparent logic and reason. In other words, the paranoid person can present seemingly justified evidence to explain his or her suspicions and beliefs.

There can be varying levels of paranoid functioning ranging from relatively mild levels of distrust of other people, to extreme, irrational distrust of others. Such feelings may escalate to the point where the person acts irrationally, feels he or she is being pursued by unseen enemies, and eventually takes action against the perceived enemies or pursuers. A paranoid person is delusional, believing people are hostile, are intent upon doing harm, and harbor ill will toward the person so affected.

Paxil. A latest-generation antidepressant medication capable of blocking the reuptake of serotonin in the brain, thereby raising the levels of serotonin. It's called a selective serotonin reuptake inhibitor, or SSRI. Serotonin has the effect of lessening both depression and anxiety. The medication can be very effective in treating depression and in modulating anxiety and panic.

Paxil and other medications in its class have been approved by the FDA for treating the symptoms of depression, panic disorder, obsessive-compulsive disorder, generalized anxiety disorder, social anxiety, phobias, and post-traumatic stress disorder. Other medications similar to Paxil include Prozac, Zoloft, Luvox, Lexapro, and Celexa.

Some newer antidepressants act not only by raising serotonin levels but also by raising the amount of norepinephrine in the brain. They're called serotonin norepinephrine reuptake inhibitors, or SNRIs. The most frequently used are Cymbalta, Effexor, and Pristiq.

personality. An enduring pattern of inner experience and behavior with which a person interacts throughout life. Generally, it is permanently set by the end of adolescence.

personality disorder. An enduring pattern of inner experience and behavior that deviates from cultural expectations, is inflexible and pervasive, has its onset in adolescence or early adulthood, is stable over time, and leads to distress or impairment in occupational and social functioning. There are different types of personality disorders: paranoid, schizoid, schizotypal, dramatic antisocial, borderline, histrionic, narcissistic, anxious, avoidant, dependent, and obsessive-compulsive. Of course, these are generalized labels, and we may see elements of one personality disorder mixed with those of another.

phantom limb. The sensation that an amputated limb is still attached to the body and is moving appropriately with other body parts. Approximately 60 to 80 percent of individuals with an amputation experience phantom sensations in the missing limb, and the majority of the sensations are painful. Various reasons have been proposed to account for this phenomenon, ranging from irritation of the severed nerves to intact representation of the missing limb in the brain. Willie Mae E. experienced phantom limb pain after having lost her leg when she jumped in front of an oncoming train. (See "When a Patient Knows More Than the Doctor.")

pharmacotherapy. Treatment of psychiatric symptoms with medication. It is often used in conjunction with psychotherapy and research has shown best therapeutic results are usually obtained when both psychotherapy and pharmacotherapy are used in conjunction with each other. Often symptoms may be smothered by medication, and psychotherapy helps the patient understand the reasons the symptoms arose. Such understanding (insight) may help the person avoid developing symptoms in the future. When symptoms abate, the medication can be slowly tapered and then discontinued.

Recent evidence seems to suggest there may be biomarkers within the brain indicating whether a specific patient will respond better to pharmacotherapy or psychotherapy. One day soon we may be able to quickly scan a patient's brain with an MRI or a PET scan, check the brain activity "fingerprint," and select an antidepressant or psychotherapy accordingly. Other research points to finding measurable biological indices to determine which *specific* antidepressant medication will be best suited for a particular patient.

placebo. A neutral substance having positive effects because of a patient's perception or belief it is beneficial rather than as a result of an active ingredient. It may be an inactive ingredient or a preparation used as a control in an experiment to determine the effectiveness of a drug. A placebo may also be an actual medication used to treat a condition but is administered in so *low a dose* as to have no "real" therapeutic effect. Rather, the person receiving the medication *perceives* and *believes* the medication is helping and therefore experiences relief from symptoms.

The placebo effect points out the importance of the mind's perception of pain or other symptoms—physical and mental. Barbara C.'s therapist thought she was experiencing a placebo effect when her medication dose was lowered to a less-than-therapeutic level, and she was still obsession- and compulsion-free. (See "A Dirty Little Secret.")

post-traumatic stress disorder (PTSD). An anxiety disorder following exposure to an extreme traumatic stressor that is generally agreed to be *beyond the range* of usual human experience. The stressor is experienced with an overwhelming sense of fear and terror, and often, with an impending sense of annihilation.

Traumatic stressors capable of evoking the disorder include wartime combat, riots, rape, explosions and collapse of physical structures (such as happened on 9/11), surviving an airplane crash, train derailment, severe automobile accidents with deaths or serious injuries, muggings or rapes with a threat to the life or bodily integrity of the victim, witnessing the violent death of a loved one, industrial accidents with death and injury, incarceration in a concentration camp (as occurred with Nathan B.), *learning* of the *violent* death of a loved one (also Nathan B.), and other extremely traumatic events.

During my psychiatric career, I consulted with and evaluated more than three hundred survivors of the September 11, 2001, terrorist attack on New York City's World Trade Center. Most suffered from severe forms of PTSD after having made their way down fifty or more crowded, smoke-filled stairwells, choking and coughing, and after having seen the bodies of those who had jumped from the highest floors after being trapped in the burning towers.

PTSD is *not* caused by ordinary incidents such as minor automobile accidents (fender benders), tripping on a sidewalk, or other unpleasant events that may occur in everyday life.

The disorder is characterized by intrusive thoughts and recollections of the trauma, along with the feelings of terror approximating the feelings experienced when the traumatic event occurred (often termed *flashbacks*). Also present may be recurrent nightmares, sleeplessness, generalized anxiety, fear when faced with situations similar to the traumatic event, and a wish to avoid any experience symbolizing, representing, or approximating the traumatic event. Exposure to such a stimulus can set off a panic attack. (I once treated a Vietnam veteran with PTSD who traveled by airplane to Florida. After exiting the Miami airport, he suddenly felt the heat and humidity, and saw a grove of palm trees. He was overcome by a full-fledged panic attack since these stimuli were reminiscent of his wartime experience in Vietnam.)

Post-traumatic stress disorder may also involve numbing of feelings, a lessened capacity for love or intimacy, and a foreshortened sense of the future.

preponderance of evidence. The burden of proof required in a civil lawsuit to show that its version of facts is *more likely than not the correct version.* This contrasts with *beyond a reasonable doubt*, which is a more rigorous test of evidence required in a criminal matter.

psychiatry. The medical specialty dealing with disorders of thinking, feeling, and behavior. A psychiatrist is a medical doctor who has undergone an internship followed by a three-year psychiatric residency. A psychiatrist can do psychotherapy, prescribe medication, and when necessary, administer ECT (electroconvulsive therapy).

psychology. The study of the human mind and its functioning. A psychologist has a graduate degree in psychology. Psychologists can do psychotherapy, psychological testing, and psychological evaluations, and are fully qualified mental health professionals.

psychosis. An acute or a chronic mental state marked by loss of contact with reality, and disorganized speech and behavior, and often accompanied by hallucinations or delusions, especially in certain mental illnesses, such as schizophrenia.

psychotropic medications. Sometimes called psychoactive drugs. Medications that affect the central nervous system, especially various sites within the brain. Such drugs can cause changes in feelings, perception, thinking, or behavior. A common misconception is that all psychotropic drugs are illegal, such as angel dust and/or marijuana. However, caffeine is a psychotropic drug, as is alcohol. Psychotropic drugs can be hallucinogens (like LSD), antipsychotics (like Risperdal), depressants (alcohol and sedatives), stimulants (amphetamines and caffeine), and antidepressants (Prozac and Effexor, among others).

resistance. A phenomenon often encountered in psychotherapy in which the patient either directly or indirectly opposes changing behavior. It can involve evading or even refusing to discuss, remember, or think about experiences, thoughts, or feelings that are upsetting or that force the patient to confront unpleasant truths, fantasies, or impulses he or she would rather avoid acknowledging.

schizophrenia. A group of psychiatric disorders thought to be associated with chemical imbalance in the brain, usually characterized by psychotic behavior including delusions, hallucinations, withdrawal from reality, and disorganized patterns of thinking and speech. There are various types of schizophrenia with different presenting signs and symptoms and different prognoses. (The man posing as Dr. Boris Papalini suffered from schizophrenia, as did Willie Mae E.)

shame. A feeling that arises due to having violated some standard of behavior. It can be viewed as an inner condemnation of the *self*. Generally speaking, shame is a feeling of social embarrassment for having done something wrong or perceived to be wrong in the *presence of others*. While many people use *shame* and *guilt* interchangeably, they are distinctly separate. There are a number of theoretical distinctions between these feeling states, but for practical reasons, guilt refers to a sense of having failed to live up to an internalized standard, while shame relates to a sense of having not lived up to certain standards in the presence of others.

Guilt and shame can be experienced simultaneously. For instance, a biting comment made toward someone at a dinner party might evoke guilt in the person who was hurtful at the expense of someone else. The person making the comment could also experience shame, since the comment was made in the presence of others who disapprove of such behavior.

sign. The physical manifestation of injury, illness, or disease. A sign is an *objective* indication of a disease, such as an enlarged liver, an irregular heartbeat, a swollen gland, or a fever. In psychiatry, a sign may be a patient crying, pacing, wringing his or her hands, excessively sweating, stammering, talking in a tremulous voice, or other actions that objectively indicate a disorder. Other signs of mental disturbance include disordered language, disheveled appearance, trembling, severe aggression toward others, bizarre gestures, and catatonic posture, among others.

somatization. The tendency to experience psychological distress in the form of bodily symptoms and to seek medical help for them. Typically, this is a defense against acknowledging unacceptable or painful thoughts, feelings, conflicts, or memories. (Mary C. in "A Deeper Cut" was a patient who used somatization.)

straitjacket. See **camisole**.

subdural hematoma. A condition that involves bleeding from a vein into the space between the dura (the brain cover) and the brain itself. This space into which the blood accumulates is called the subdural space. If the hematoma (collection of blood) puts increased pressure on the brain, neurological abnormalities including slurred speech, impaired gait, and dizziness may result, progressing to coma and death. Subdural hematomas are different from epidural hematomas, which involve arterial bleeding from a vessel above the dura mater (the covering of the brain). Epidural hematomas are more dangerous since arterial bleeding is more rapid than venous bleeding and can quickly cause a swelling, putting great pressure on the brain, which is confined by the surrounding skull.

survivor's guilt. Sometimes called guilt of the survivor. A condition that may occur when a person irrationally feels he or she has done "wrong" by surviving a traumatic event in which others died.

It is seen with some frequency among people who have survived concentration camps, natural disasters, wartime combat, and other catastrophic situations. The propensity to develop survivor's guilt depends on a person's psychologic makeup and the circumstances of the traumatic event. It is often seen as a significant component of post-traumatic stress disorder. It can also result in a full-fledged state of clinical depression. (See "King of the Puerto Ricans.")

symptom. A subjective sensation reported by a patient, but one that cannot be verified by objective examination. Feeling tired, dizzy, or nauseous and experiencing pain are symptoms. Psychiatrically, a symptom may involve feeling helpless, overwhelmed, or saddened by a situation. It is a symptom when there are no verifiable or objective signs or indications of inner distress. A symptom may be accompanied by a sign, such as when a depressed person becomes tearful, begins wringing hands and pacing, or develops insomnia with early-morning awakening, or when someone complains of feeling hot and when his or her temperature is taken is found to have a fever.

transcranial magnetic stimulation (TMS). A procedure using magnetic fields to stimulate the brain to improve symptoms of depression. It may be tried when other depression treatments have failed. The procedure uses an electromagnetic coil on the scalp, producing electric currents to stimulate nerve cells in the amygdala, the region of the brain controlling mood.

tricyclic antidepressants. Introduced in the 1950s, among the earliest antidepressant medications developed and an important advance in psychiatric treatment. They're effective but have generally been replaced by the newer generation of antidepressants, SSRIs and SNRIs. Tricyclic antidepressants remain a good option for some people. In certain cases, they relieve depression when other medications have failed. In fact, certain people respond far better to one specific medication (whether it's a tricyclic or an SSRI) than others, implicating individual biological pathways and mechanisms in different people.

It's thought tricyclic medications ease depression by affecting naturally occurring chemical messengers (neurotransmitters such as serotonin, epinephrine, and dopamine) used to communicate between brain cells by blocking the absorption (reuptake) of these neurotransmitters. The blockade makes the neurotransmitters more available, helping brain cells send and receive messages. This, in turn, boosts mood. Most antidepressants work by changing the levels of one or more neurotransmitters.

The most common tricyclic antidepressants used were Elavil, Tofranil, Pamelor, Vivactil, and Surmontil. These medications have many side effects, which often cause patients to discontinue use. In addition, an overdose can cause serious and sometimes fatal complications. This is generally not the case for the later generation of medications, the SSRIs and SNRIs.

word salad. A condition in which a person attempts to communicate an idea, but instead words and phrases appear random and unrelated, and come out in an incoherent sequence. Often the person is unaware that he or she did not make sense. Word salad may occur in people with dementia or schizophrenia, or after a severe brain injury or stroke.

References

King of the Puerto Ricans

Andreasen, Nancy C. "Acute and Delayed Posttraumatic Stress Disorders: A History and Some Issues." *American Journal of Psychiatry* 161, no. 8 (2004): 1321–23.

Brewin, Chris. *Posttraumatic Stress Disorder: Malady or Myth?* New Haven: Yale University Press, 2003.

A Helping Hand

Blair, R. "The Emergence of Psychopathy: Implications for the Neuropsychological Approach to Developmental Disorders." *Cognition* 101, no. 2 (2006): 414–42.

Kernberg, Otto F. *Borderline Conditions and Pathological Narcissism.* New York: J. Aronson, 1975.

Krishnan, Vaishnav, and Eric J. Nestler. "The Molecular Neurobiology of Depression." *Nature* 455, no. 7215 (2008): 894–902.

Oquendo, Maria A. "Impulsive versus Planned Suicide Attempts." *Journal of Clinical Psychiatry* 76, no. 3 (2015): 293–94.

Sareen, Jitender, Brian J. Cox, Tracie O. Afifi, et al. "Anxiety Disorders and Risk for Suicidal Ideation and Suicide Attempts." *Archives of General Psychiatry* 62, no. 11 (2005): 1249–57.

Simon, Robert I. "Passive Suicidal Ideation: Still a High-Risk Clinical Scenario." *Current Psychiatry* 13, no. 3 (March 2014): 13–15.

Simon, Robert I., and Robert E. Hales. *The American Psychiatric Publishing Textbook of Suicide Assessment and Management.* Washington, DC: American Psychiatric Publishing, 2012.

The Head Doctor

Simons, Richard C., and Herbert Pardes. *Understanding Human Behavior in Health and Illness.* 2nd ed. Baltimore: Williams & Wilkins, 1981.

Waitzkin, H. "Doctor-Patient Communication: Clinical Implications of Social Scientific Research." *Journal of the American Medical Association* 252, no. 17 (1984): 2441–46.

Baptism by Fire

American Psychiatric Association. *Diagnostic and Statistical Manual of Mental Disorders: DSM-5.* Washington, DC: American Psychiatric Publishing, 2013.

Kubler-Ross, Elizabeth. *On Death and Dying.* New York: Scribner, 1969.

New York State Office of Mental Health. *Rights of Inpatients in New York State Office of Mental Health Psychiatric Centers.* New York: Office of Mental Health, modified November 9, 2012, http://www.omh.ny.gov/omhweb/patientrights/inpatient_rts .htm.

A Man of Means

New York State Office of Mental Health. *Rights of Inpatients in New York State Office of Mental Health Psychiatric Centers.* New York: Office of Mental Health, modified November 9, 2012.

NY Mental Hygiene Law, §§ 9.01, 9.05, 9.31, and 9.37 (2015).

A Dirty Little Secret

American Psychiatric Association. *Diagnostic and Statistical Manual of Mental Disorders: DSM-5.* Washington, DC: American Psychiatric Publishing, 2013.

Sadock, Benjamin J., and Virginia A. Sadock. *Kaplan & Sadock's Comprehensive Textbook of Psychiatry.* 9th ed. Philadelphia: Lippincott Williams & Wilkins, 2009.

Simons, Richard C., and Herbert Pardes. *Understanding Human Behavior in Health and Illness.* 2nd ed. Baltimore: Williams & Wilkins, 1981.

When a Patient Knows More Than the Doctor

American Psychiatric Association. *Diagnostic and Statistical Manual of Mental Disorders: DSM-5.* Washington, DC: American Psychiatric Publishing, 2013.

Sadock, Benjamin J., and Virginia A. Sadock. *Kaplan & Sadock's Comprehensive Textbook of Psychiatry*. 9th ed. Philadelphia: Lippincott Williams & Wilkins, 2009.

Simon, Robert I., and Liza H. Gold. *The American Psychiatric Publishing Textbook of Forensic Psychiatry*. Washington, DC: American Psychiatric Publishing, 2010.

Dr. Boris Papalini

Barbanel, J. "Suspect in Slaying Was Treated at Bellevue." *New York Times*, January 12, 1989.

Brunton, Laurence, Bruce Chabner, and Bjorn Knollman. *Goodman and Gilman's The Pharmacological Basis of Therapeutics*. New York: McGraw-Hill, 2011.

McKee, J. "Lack of Mental-Health Treatment Options Clogs Criminal Justice System." *Helena Independent Record*, October 2, 2007.

Nocera, J. "For the Mentally Ill, It's Worse." *New York Times*, January 24, 2014.

Sadock, Benjamin J., and Virginia A. Sadock. *Kaplan & Sadock's Comprehensive Textbook of Psychiatry*. 9th ed. Philadelphia: Lippincott Williams & Wilkins, 2009.

Steadman, Henry J., Fred C. Osher, Pamela Clark Robbins, Brian Case, and Steven Samuels. "Prevalence of Serious Mental Illness among Jail Inmates." *Psychiatric Services* 60, no. 6 (2009): 761–65.

Off the Wall

Black's Law Dictionary. 10th ed. Thomson West, 2014.

Silver, Jonathan M., Stuart C. Yudofsky, and Robert E. Hales. *Neuropsychiatry of Traumatic Brain Injury*. Washington, DC: American Psychiatric Publishing, 1994.

Strub, Richard L., and F. William Black. *Neurobehavioral Disorders: A Clinical Approach*. Philadelphia: Davis, 1988.

Yudofsky, Stuart C., and Robert E. Hales. *The American Psychiatric Publishing Textbook of Neuropsychiatry and Behavioral Neurosciences*. 5th ed. Washington, DC: American Psychiatric Publishing, 2007.

The Family and Me

Black's Law Dictionary. 10th ed. Thomson West, 2014.

McFadden, Robert D. "Galante and 2 Shot to Death in a Brooklyn Restaurant." *New York Times*, July 13, 1979.

Simon, Robert I., and Liza H. Gold. *The American Psychiatric Publishing Textbook of Forensic Psychiatry*. Washington, DC: American Psychiatric Publishing, 2010.

Vitaly Tarasoff et al. v. The Regents of the University of California et al., S.F. No. 23042 Supreme Court of California, 17 Cal. 3d 425, 551 P.2d 334, 131 Cal. Rptr. 14, 1976 Cal. LEXIS 297, 83 A.L.R.3d 1166 (July 1, 1976).

A Deeper Cut

American Psychiatric Association. *Diagnostic and Statistical Manual of Mental Disorders: DSM-5*. Washington, DC: American Psychiatric Publishing, 2013.

Hales, Robert E., Stuart C. Yudofsky, and Glen O. Gabbard. *Essentials of Psychiatry*. Washington, DC: American Psychiatric Publishing, 2010.

Sadock, Benjamin J., and Virginia A. Sadock. *Kaplan & Sadock's Comprehensive Textbook of Psychiatry*. Philadelphia: Lippincott Williams & Wilkins, 2009.

A Brief Last Word

Brunk, Doug. "Neuroimaging Making Inroads as a Diagnostic Tool." *Clinical Psychiatry News* 43, no. 4 (April 2015).

Brunton, Laurence, Bruce Chabner, and Bjorn Knollman. *Goodman and Gilman's The Pharmacological Basis of Therapeutics*. New York: McGraw-Hill, 2011.

Friedman, Richard A. "Brought on by Darkness, Disorder Needs Light." *New York Times*, December 18, 2007.

Mueller, Sophia, Danhong Wang, Ruiqi Pan, Daphne J. Holt, and Hesheng Liu. "Abnormalities in Hemispheric Specialization of Caudate Nucleus Connectivity in Schizophrenia." *JAMA Psychiatry* 72, no. 6 (2015): 552.

Ross, David A., Michael J. Travis, and Melissa R. Arbuckle. "The Future of Psychiatry as Clinical Neuroscience." *JAMA Psychiatry* 72, no. 5 (2015): 413.

Shorter, Edward. *A History of Psychiatry: From the Era of the Asylum to the Age of Prozac.* New York: Wiley, 1998.

Stratton, John, Kent A. Kiehl, and Robert E. Hanlon. "The Neurobiology of Psychopathy." *Psychiatric Annals* 45, no. 4 (2015): 186–94.

Wheeler, Anne L., Michele Wessa, Phillip R. Szeszko, et al. "Further Neuroimaging Evidence for the Deficit Subtype of Schizophrenia." *JAMA Psychiatry* 72, no. 5 (2015): 446.

Suggested Reading

These suggestions are by no means exhaustive, but for the reader who wishes to learn more about psychiatry, psychology, mental illness, and various treatments, they provide a good foundation.

DSM-5 by the American Psychiatric Association. This tome is not easy reading. It's a compendium describing all known mental disorders. It's not written for the reader to gain an understanding of mental illness, but rather, it is a manual for classifying and describing the known mental disorders. It provides an overview of the range of conditions currently viewed as pathologic. The word *current* applies since the manual is revised every few years to reflect new findings and trends, and occasionally, to accommodate social realities. It's often referred to in courtroom proceedings as the bible of psychiatry. I've often characterized it as cookbook psychiatry, but it can be valuable for its descriptions of mental disorders: the age of onset, course, epidemiologic characteristics, and other descriptive aspects of these conditions.

Listening with the Third Ear by Dr. Theodor Reik. This is an older book written by an esteemed psychologist who was a student of Freud's. Dr. Reik describes important aspects of mental and emotional functioning using a psychoanalytic/psychodynamic approach. He writes in an engaging and entertaining way, using vivid case histories and examples to make many important points about the human mind. He also emphasizes the importance of using self-knowledge to understand his patients. It's really a fun read.

Kaplan & Sadock's Comprehensive Textbook of Psychiatry, edited by Benjamin J. Sadock and Virginia Alcott Sadock. This massive, two-volume set has long been considered the cornerstone textbook in the field of psychiatry. The ninth edition provides information about neural science, genetics, neuropsychiatry, and psychopharmacotherapy. More than five hundred contributors provide up-to-date information in every area of psychiatry and mental health. It is so filled with information, it can be overwhelming and isn't for the faint of heart. But for the serious student, it's a fine reference book. Warning: it's very expensive—$300 in hardcover—but costs much less if purchased used from Amazon or in bookstores. Also available is ***Kaplan & Sadock's Synopsis of Psychiatry***, which costs less than $100 and has plenty of information for the general reader. This, too, is available on Amazon as a used book and is quite inexpensive.

Understanding Human Behavior in Health and Illness, edited by Richard C. Simons and Herbert Pardes. This wonderful textbook was originally written for medical students. In clear, easily digestible form, it provides a wealth of information about nearly every aspect of mental health—diagnosis; treatment; genetic, social, and environmental factors—and addresses virtually every area of psychiatry, psychology, and allied fields. Geared toward laypeople, it's the most accessible textbook of those mentioned. It's available on Amazon in both new and used editions.

The First Encounter: The Beginnings in Psychotherapy by William A. Console, Richard C. Simons, and Mark Rubinstein. This book has eye-opening dissections of five initial interviews conducted by Dr. William Console, a masterful clinician—a psychiatrist and psychoanalyst—and an astute explorer of the human mind. The volume demonstrates many principles of psychiatry, psychology, and psychoanalysis, and an array of interviewing techniques. It illustrates the incredible wealth of information that can be obtained in the very first meeting with a patient. The book is available on Amazon.

Acknowledgments

Any author's work is the final common pathway of a lifetime of learning, inspiration, motivation, and collaboration.

I owe more than I can express to the thousands of patients I saw over the years—in various hospitals and clinics, and in my private practice, whether for treatment or consultations. Many others were seen for forensic purposes involving litigation, competency matters regarding contracts, or testamentary capacity. Others were seen for workers' compensation evaluations, or for assessments at the request of the New York State and Connecticut Bureaus of Disability Determinations.

No matter the venue in which I saw them, patients helped me learn about psychiatry and psychotherapy, and taught me valuable lessons about life, and myself, as well. And some provided the case histories and material for the stories in this book.

My education as a psychiatrist was nurtured by the efforts of three outstanding teachers to whom I shall always remain indebted: Dr. William Console, Dr. Richard Simons, and Dr. Warren Tanenbaum.

My forensic experience was enhanced by contact with a stellar group of trial attorneys, judges, and commissioners with whom I worked over the years, whether in court or at depositions, hearings, or other legal and social venues. I owe them more than I can say. Among many things I learned was a simple maxim: in the courtroom, it was never my job to be either an adversary or an advocate. My task was simple: to provide the clinical truth as I understood it, no matter which side retained my services.

As for my writing life, Kristen Weber, a fabulous editor, has helped me enormously. She has been my mentor and encouraged me to write both fiction and nonfiction.

Sharon Goldinger, Skye Wentworth, Victoria Colotta, Penina Lopez, Linda Seeley, and Tracy Topalu have helped my efforts in many ways.

My interface with writers over the years sharpened my writing ability and taught me more than I can articulate. Thank you to every writer I've interviewed, or with whom I shared an author panel, a telephone conversation, a lunch, or a dinner. Every contact with these writers has been a learning experience and a pleasure. I look forward to many more interviews and discussions with them.

I owe a special word of thanks to Dr. Donna Sutter.

My wife, Linda, has always been my strongest advocate and is blessed with infinite patience and wisdom. She's my editor in chief and the CEO of my life. Without her I would probably never have written anything.

About the Author

After graduating from NYU with a degree in business admin-istration, Mark Rubinstein served in the US Army as a field medic tending to paratroopers of the 82nd Airborne Division at Fort Bragg, North Carolina. After discharge from the army, he returned to NYU to complete courses in the premedical sciences. He gained admission to medical school. After becoming a phy-sician, he undertook a psychiatric residency and developed an interest in forensic psychiatry. Over the years he testified as an expert witness in many jury trials, depositions, arbitrations, and hearings.

He was an attending psychiatrist on hospital wards, in a psychiatric emergency room, and in various outpatient psychi-atric clinics, including the South Beach Psychiatric Center. He was an attending psychiatrist at Kings County Hospital and New York Presbyterian Hospital's Payne Whitney Clinic and a clinical assistant professor of psychiatry at Downstate Medical Center of the State University of New York and then at Cornell University Medical School. He taught psychiatric interns, resi-dents, psychologists, psychiatric nurses, and social workers while practicing psychiatry in private practices in New York City and Connecticut.

Before turning to fiction, he coauthored five nonfiction, self-help books for the general public. His first novel, *Mad Dog House*, was a finalist for the 2012 IndieFab Book of the Year Awards in the Thriller and Suspense category, and his novel *Mad Dog Justice* was a finalist for the 2014 IndieFab Book of the Year Awards in the Thriller and Suspense category. His novella *The Foot Soldier* won the Silver award in Popular Fiction in the 2014 Benjamin Franklin Book Awards, and his novella *Return to Sandara* won the 2015 Gold IPPY Award for Suspense/Thriller Fiction. His most recent novel, *The Lovers' Tango*, won the Gold award in Popular Fiction in the 2016 Benjamin Franklin Book Awards. He contributes regularly to the *Huffington Post* and *Psychology Today*.

You can contact Mark via the following:

Website: http://markrubinstein-author.com

Twitter: @mrubinsteinCT

E-mail: author.mark.rubinstein@gmail.com